PEJMAN HAJBABAIE

Understanding Stomach Diseases

First edition

This book was professionally typeset on Reedsy.
Find out more at reedsy.com

Contents

1

Chapter 1: Anatomy and Physiology of the Stomach

Gross Anatomy of the Stomach

The gross anatomy of the stomach is a vital aspect of understanding its role in the digestive system. The stomach is a muscular, hollow organ located between the oesophagus and the small intestine. It is divided into four main regions: the cardia, fundus, body, and pylorus. Each of these areas serves a distinct function in the digestive process, contributing to the breakdown of food and the preparation of nutrients for absorption.

The cardia is the section where the oesophagus connects to the stomach. This area is crucial as it contains the lower oesophageal sphincter, which prevents the backflow of stomach contents into the oesophagus. Just above the cardia is the fundus, which serves as a storage area for undigested food and gases released during digestion. The shape of the fundus can vary depending on the amount of food in the stomach, expanding as needed.

Following the fundus is the body of the stomach, which is the largest region. This section plays a central role in mixing and churning food with gastric juices, which contain hydrochloric acid and digestive enzymes. The body's muscular walls contract rhythmically, aiding in the mechanical breakdown of food particles into a semi-liquid substance known as chyme. This process is essential for effective digestion and nutrient absorption.

The pylorus, located at the distal end of the stomach, connects to the small intestine. It is surrounded by a thick ring of muscle known as the pyloric sphincter, which regulates the passage of chyme into the duodenum. This sphincter ensures that food is released in a controlled manner, allowing for optimal digestion and preventing the rapid passage of food into the intestines, which can hinder nutrient absorption.

Understanding the gross anatomy of the stomach not only provides insights into its functional capabilities but also highlights the importance of each region in the digestive process. Any abnormalities or diseases affecting these areas can significantly impact digestion and overall health. Therefore, a comprehensive knowledge of the stomach's structure is essential for anyone wishing to understand stomach diseases and their implications.

Cellular Structure of the Stomach

The stomach is a complex organ that plays a crucial role in digestion. Its cellular structure is intricately designed to facilitate the breakdown of food and the absorption of nutrients. The stomach wall is composed of four main layers: the mucosa, submucosa, muscularis, and serosa, each contributing to the overall function of this vital organ.

The mucosa is the innermost layer, lined with specialised epithelial cells that secrete gastric juices. These juices contain hydrochloric acid and digestive enzymes, which are essential for breaking down food particles. The mucosa also contains gastric pits, which house the gastric glands responsible for producing these secretions. This layer is crucial for the initial stages of digestion.

Beneath the mucosa lies the submucosa, a layer rich in blood vessels, nerves, and connective tissue. This layer supports the mucosa and provides it with the necessary nutrients and oxygen. The presence of nerve endings in the submucosa is vital for regulating gastric secretions and ensuring the smooth functioning of digestive processes.

The muscularis layer consists of smooth muscle fibres arranged in three distinct layers: an inner oblique layer, a middle circular layer, and an outer longitudinal layer. This arrangement enables the stomach to perform powerful contractions, mixing food with gastric juices and propelling it towards the intestines. These muscular movements, known as peristalsis, are essential for effective digestion.

Finally, the outermost layer, the serosa, is a protective covering that reduces friction between the stomach and surrounding organs. It plays a crucial role in maintaining the integrity of the stomach structure. Understanding the cellular architecture of the stomach is fundamental to comprehending its function and the various diseases that can affect it, thus paving the way for better diagnostic and treatment strategies.

Hormonal Regulation of Gastric Function

Hormonal regulation plays a crucial role in managing gastric function, influencing processes such as digestion and gastric motility. The stomach produces several hormones, including gastrin, ghrelin, and somatostatin, each of which has distinct functions that contribute to the overall digestive process. Gastrin, for example, stimulates gastric acid secretion and promotes the growth of the gastric mucosa, ensuring that the stomach can effectively break down food.

Ghrelin, often referred to as the 'hunger hormone', is produced in the stomach and signals the brain to stimulate appetite. Its levels rise before meals and decrease after eating, thus playing a pivotal role in meal initiation and energy balance. This regulatory mechanism is essential for maintaining proper nutritional intake and can impact overall health if disrupted.

Somatostatin, another significant hormone, acts to inhibit the release of gastrin and other digestive hormones. By doing so, it plays a balancing role in gastric function, preventing excessive gastric acid secretion and ensuring the stomach does not become overwhelmed during digestion. This regulatory feedback is vital for the smooth operation of the digestive system.

The interplay between these hormones is complex and can be influenced by various factors, including stress, diet, and overall health. Disruptions in hormonal levels can lead to gastric disorders, such as gastritis or peptic ulcers, highlighting the importance of hormonal balance in maintaining gastric health. Understanding these mechanisms is crucial for developing effective treatments for stomach diseases.

In conclusion, hormonal regulation is fundamental to gastric function, affecting everything from appetite to digestion. By understanding how these hormones interact and their effects on the stomach, we can better appreciate the intricate workings of our digestive system and the potential impacts of hormonal imbalances on health. This knowledge is essential for both medical professionals and individuals seeking to understand stomach diseases more comprehensively.

Acid Secretion and Protection

The stomach is a remarkable organ, primarily responsible for digesting food. It achieves this through the secretion of gastric acid, primarily hydrochloric acid, which plays a crucial role in breaking down food particles and activating digestive enzymes. This acidic environment is essential for optimal digestion, as it helps to kill harmful bacteria that may enter the stomach with food. Understanding how acid secretion works is vital for comprehending various stomach diseases that can occur due to imbalances in this process.

Acid secretion is regulated by a complex interplay of neural and hormonal signals. The presence of food in the stomach stimulates the release of gastrin, a hormone that promotes the production of gastric acid. Additionally, the vagus nerve, which innervates the stomach, enhances acid secretion during the digestive process. This finely-tuned system ensures that the stomach maintains an appropriate level of acidity for effective digestion, but it can be disrupted by factors such as stress, diet, and certain medications.

While gastric acid is essential for digestion, it can also lead to complications if not properly regulated. Excessive acid production can result in conditions such as gastroesophageal reflux disease (GORD) and peptic ulcers, which can cause significant discomfort and damage to the stomach lining. Conversely, insufficient acid secretion may hinder proper digestion, leading to malnutrition and other gastrointestinal issues. Therefore, maintaining a balance in acid secretion is crucial for gastrointestinal health.

The stomach has its own mechanisms for protecting itself from the corrosive effects of acid. The gastric mucosa, or stomach lining, secretes a thick layer of mucus that acts as a barrier against acid. This mucus layer is essential for preventing damage to the stomach tissues. Additionally, bicarbonate ions are secreted to neutralise any excess acidity in the stomach. These protective mechanisms are vital in preventing conditions such as gastritis and ulcers, which can arise from a breakdown in this protective barrier.

In conclusion, acid secretion and protection are integral aspects of stomach function. A thorough understanding of these processes can help individuals recognise symptoms of stomach diseases and seek appropriate treatment. By appreciating the delicate balance between acid production and protective mechanisms, one can gain insight into maintaining gastrointestinal health and addressing potential disorders effectively.

Neural Regulation and the Enteric Nervous System

The enteric nervous system (ENS) is often referred to as the "second brain" due to its complexity and autonomy. It is a vast network of neurons embedded within the walls of the gastrointestinal tract, enabling it to operate independently of the central nervous system. This system plays a crucial role in regulating digestion, including the coordination of muscle contractions and the secretion of digestive enzymes. Understanding the ENS is essential for grasping how various stomach diseases can affect overall gastrointestinal function.

Neural regulation within the ENS involves intricate communication between neurons, glial cells, and the gastrointestinal smooth muscle. These cells work together to process information about the state of the gut, responding to stimuli such as food presence and chemical signals. This communication ensures that the digestive process is efficient and well-coordinated. Disruptions in this neural regulation can lead to conditions such as irritable bowel syndrome and functional dyspepsia, which manifest in various gastrointestinal symptoms.

Moreover, the ENS is influenced by the microbiome, the diverse community of microorganisms residing in the gut. These microbes can interact with the nervous system, sending signals that affect mood, appetite, and digestion. This relationship underscores the importance of maintaining a healthy gut microbiome, as imbalances can contribute to digestive disorders and affect the ENS's ability to regulate stomach function effectively.

In addition to its role in digestion, the ENS is also involved in the gut-brain axis, a communication network linking the gastrointestinal tract to the brain. This connection illustrates how stress and emotional states can influence gut health and vice versa. Disorders such as anxiety and depression have been shown to affect gastrointestinal function, highlighting the importance of a holistic approach to treating stomach diseases that considers both physical and mental health.

In conclusion, the neural regulation of the enteric nervous system is fundamental to understanding stomach diseases. By exploring the complex interactions between the ENS, gut microbiome, and the brain, researchers can develop more effective treatments for gastrointestinal disorders. As our knowledge of the ENS expands, so too does our ability to address the myriad challenges posed by stomach diseases, ultimately improving patient outcomes and quality of life.

2

Chapter 2: How the Stomach Works in Digestion

Mechanical and Chemical Digestion

Mechanical digestion and chemical digestion are two essential processes that occur in the stomach, playing a vital role in the overall digestion of food. Mechanical digestion involves the physical breakdown of food into smaller pieces. This process begins in the mouth with chewing and continues in the stomach, where muscular contractions help to further break down the food, mixing it with gastric juices. These actions ensure that food is adequately prepared for the next stage of digestion.

Chemical digestion, on the other hand, involves the breakdown of food at a molecular level through the action of enzymes and acids. In the stomach, gastric acid, primarily hydrochloric acid, activates digestive enzymes that begin the process of breaking down proteins into smaller peptides. This chemical transformation is crucial for nutrient absorption, as it converts complex food substances into simpler molecules that can be easily absorbed by the body.

The interplay between mechanical and chemical digestion is significant in ensuring optimal digestive health. For instance, if mechanical digestion is insufficient, larger food particles may not be broken down adequately, leading to a reduced surface area for enzymes to act upon during chemical digestion. This can result in incomplete digestion, causing discomfort and potential stomach diseases.

Furthermore, various factors can influence the efficiency of these digestive processes. For example, stress can affect the muscular contractions that facilitate mechanical digestion, while certain medications can alter the acidity of gastric juices, impacting chemical digestion. Understanding these factors is crucial for maintaining digestive health and preventing stomach-related issues.

In conclusion, both mechanical and chemical digestion are fundamental to the digestive process. They work in tandem to ensure that food is adequately broken down for nutrient absorption. A comprehensive understanding of these processes is essential for recognising how disturbances can lead to stomach diseases, emphasising the importance of digestive health in overall well-being.

Stomach Emptying and Coordination with Small Bowel

The process of stomach emptying is a vital aspect of digestion, playing a crucial role in how food is processed before entering the small bowel. This coordination between the stomach and the small intestine is essential for efficient digestion and nutrient absorption. After food is ingested, the stomach begins to break it down through mechanical and chemical means, creating a semi-liquid substance known as chyme. This chyme is then gradually released into the small bowel, where further digestion and absorption occur.

The rate at which the stomach empties its contents is influenced by several factors, including the type of food consumed, hormonal signals, and nervous system responses. For instance, high-fat meals tend to slow down the emptying process, allowing for more thorough digestion. In contrast, liquid foods may pass through the stomach more quickly. Hormones such as gastrin and cholecystokinin play a significant role in regulating these processes, ensuring that the stomach and small bowel work in harmony.

Coordination between the stomach and small bowel is also critical for preventing gastrointestinal complications. If the stomach empties too quickly, it can lead to conditions such as dumping syndrome, where undigested food moves rapidly into the small intestine. Conversely, delayed stomach emptying, known as gastroparesis, can result in bloating, nausea, and other digestive issues. Understanding these conditions helps in diagnosing and managing various stomach diseases effectively.

Additionally, the interplay between gastric motility and small bowel function is essential for maintaining optimal digestive health. The small bowel relies on a steady influx of chyme to facilitate the digestive process and nutrient absorption. Any disruption in this coordination can lead to malabsorption and other health issues. Therefore, healthcare professionals often assess both stomach emptying and small bowel function when evaluating patients with gastrointestinal complaints.

In conclusion, the relationship between stomach emptying and small bowel coordination is complex yet vital for proper digestion. Awareness of how these two systems interact aids in understanding stomach diseases and their management. By focusing on the factors that influence this process, individuals can better appreciate the importance of digestive health and seek appropriate care when necessary.

Stomach's Role in Nutrient Absorption and Vitamin B12

The stomach plays a crucial role in the digestive process, serving as a reservoir for food and a site for initial digestion. Upon ingestion, food is mixed with gastric juices, which contain hydrochloric acid and digestive enzymes. This acidic environment not only helps break down food particles but also activates enzymes that are essential for nutrient absorption. Among the various nutrients that the stomach helps to process, vitamin B12 is particularly significant due to its complex absorption mechanism.

Vitamin B12, also known as cobalamin, is vital for red blood cell formation, neurological function, and DNA synthesis. However, its absorption is not a straightforward process. The stomach produces a protein called intrinsic factor, which binds to vitamin B12 and protects it from degradation as it moves through the digestive tract. This binding is crucial because, without intrinsic factor, vitamin B12 cannot be adequately absorbed in the intestines, leading to potential deficiencies.

Stomach diseases, such as atrophic gastritis and peptic ulcers, can severely impact the production of intrinsic factor. Individuals suffering from these conditions may find it challenging to absorb vitamin B12 effectively. Consequently, they may experience symptoms of deficiency, including fatigue, weakness, and neurological issues. Understanding the interplay between the stomach and nutrient absorption is essential for those with stomach ailments, as it highlights the importance of monitoring vitamin levels.

Moreover, a healthy stomach environment is necessary for the absorption of not just vitamin B12 but also other nutrients. The balance of stomach acid is pivotal; too little acid can lead to inadequate absorption of essential vitamins and minerals. Maintaining a healthy diet and seeking medical advice when experiencing gastrointestinal symptoms can aid in preserving stomach function and nutrient absorption.

In conclusion, the stomach's role in nutrient absorption, particularly in relation to vitamin B12, cannot be overstated. Awareness of how stomach conditions affect this process is vital for managing health and preventing deficiencies. For those interested in understanding stomach diseases, recognising the importance of intrinsic factor and the implications of stomach health is a key takeaway.

3

Chapter 3: Gastric Disorders – Symptoms and Signs

Dyspepsia

Dyspepsia, commonly known as indigestion, is a prevalent condition that affects many individuals, causing discomfort in the upper abdomen. Symptoms can vary widely, including bloating, nausea, and a sensation of fullness after meals. Dyspepsia can occur due to various factors, such as dietary habits, stress, or underlying medical conditions, making it essential to understand its multifaceted nature.

The causes of dyspepsia are diverse, ranging from benign issues like overeating to more serious conditions such as gastroesophageal reflux disease (GORD) or peptic ulcers. Certain foods and beverages, particularly those that are spicy, acidic, or high in fat, can exacerbate symptoms. Additionally, lifestyle factors such as smoking and excessive alcohol consumption may also contribute to the onset of dyspepsia, highlighting the importance of a balanced diet and healthy habits.

Diagnosis of dyspepsia often involves a thorough medical history and physical examination. In some cases, further investigations like endoscopy or imaging studies may be necessary to rule out more serious underlying diseases.

Understanding the patient's symptoms and triggers is crucial for effective management and treatment, which can vary depending on the underlying cause.

Treatment options for dyspepsia typically include dietary modifications, lifestyle changes, and medications to alleviate symptoms. Antacids, proton pump inhibitors, and H2-receptor antagonists are commonly prescribed to reduce stomach acid and provide relief. Moreover, addressing psychological factors through stress management techniques can also play a significant role in improving symptoms.

In conclusion, dyspepsia is a common yet complex condition that can significantly impact daily life. By understanding its causes and symptoms, individuals can take proactive steps towards managing their digestive health. Awareness of dietary choices, lifestyle habits, and when to seek medical advice is essential for effective treatment and overall well-being.

Nausea/vomiting

Nausea and vomiting are common symptoms that can arise from a variety of underlying conditions affecting the stomach and digestive system. These symptoms can be distressing and may significantly impact a person's quality of life. Understanding the potential causes of nausea and vomiting is crucial for effective management and treatment. They may be triggered by factors such as infections, motion sickness, food intolerances, or even psychological conditions like anxiety.

In many cases, nausea serves as a warning sign that something is not right within the body. It can occur as a response to irritation of the stomach lining or as a side effect of medications. Vomiting, on the other hand, is a more severe response that expels the contents of the stomach. This process can lead to dehydration and electrolyte imbalances if not managed properly, especially in vulnerable populations such as children and the elderly.

Diagnosis of the underlying cause of nausea and vomiting typically involves a comprehensive evaluation, including a detailed medical history and physical examination. In some instances, further tests such as blood tests, imaging studies, or endoscopic procedures may be necessary to determine the root cause. Identifying whether the symptoms are acute or chronic is also essential, as this can guide the treatment approach.

Treatment options for nausea and vomiting vary depending on the underlying cause. They may include dietary modifications, medications to control nausea, and hydration strategies to prevent dehydration. In cases where nausea is linked to a chronic condition, such as gastroesophageal reflux disease (GORD) or peptic ulcers, addressing the primary condition can alleviate the symptoms.

In conclusion, while nausea and vomiting are common and often temporary symptoms, they can signal more serious health issues. It is vital for individuals experiencing persistent or severe nausea and vomiting to seek medical attention. Understanding these symptoms can lead to better management strategies and improved overall health outcomes.

Early satiety

Early satiety, a condition where a person feels full after consuming only a small amount of food, can be a perplexing issue for many. It often occurs due to various underlying health conditions, including gastrointestinal disorders, hormonal imbalances, or psychological factors. This phenomenon can significantly impact an individual's nutritional intake and overall quality of life. Understanding the causes and implications of early satiety is crucial for anyone experiencing this symptom.

One common cause of early satiety is gastroparesis, a condition characterised by delayed gastric emptying. In this situation, the stomach takes longer than normal to empty its contents into the small intestine, leading to a sensation of fullness even after eating minimal amounts of food. Other gastrointestinal issues, such as peptic ulcers or certain types of tumours, may also contribute to this uncomfortable sensation. Recognising these medical conditions is essential for proper diagnosis and treatment.

Hormonal factors can also play a significant role in early satiety. Hormones like ghrelin and leptin, which regulate hunger and fullness, can become imbalanced due to various reasons, including stress or metabolic disorders. When these hormones do not function correctly, individuals may experience an abnormal feeling of fullness. This hormonal imbalance can be a complex issue requiring a comprehensive evaluation by healthcare professionals.

Psychological factors, such as anxiety and depression, can further complicate the experience of early satiety. Emotional distress can affect eating behaviours and perception of hunger, leading to a decreased desire to eat. It is essential to address these psychological components, as they may require different intervention strategies alongside medical treatment. This holistic approach ensures that all aspects of a patient's health are considered.

In summary, early satiety is a multifaceted issue that can arise from various physical and psychological conditions. Addressing this symptom requires a thorough understanding of its potential causes and an appropriate treatment plan tailored to the individual. By recognising the importance of early satiety, individuals can seek timely medical advice and improve their overall health and well-being.

Bloating and belching

Bloating and belching are common gastrointestinal issues that affect many individuals. Bloating refers to a sensation of fullness or swelling in the abdomen, often accompanied by discomfort. It can be caused by various factors, including overeating, the consumption of gas-producing foods, or underlying medical conditions. Understanding the causes of bloating is crucial for effective management and relief.

Epigastric pain

Epigastric pain, located in the upper central region of the abdomen, is a common symptom that can arise from various underlying conditions. It often presents as a sharp, burning, or dull ache and can be associated with other gastrointestinal symptoms such as nausea, bloating, and changes in appetite. Understanding the nature of this pain is crucial for both patients and healthcare providers, as it can indicate anything from benign issues to serious medical concerns.

Common causes of epigastric pain include gastritis, peptic ulcers, and gastroesophageal reflux disease (GORD). Gastritis, an inflammation of the stomach lining, can lead to discomfort and is often triggered by factors such as alcohol consumption, stress, or certain medications. Peptic ulcers, which are sores that develop on the stomach lining or the upper part of the small intestine, can cause significant pain and may require medical intervention if they become severe.

In addition to these conditions, epigastric pain can also be a sign of more serious issues, such as pancreatitis or even cardiac problems. Pancreatitis, an inflammation of the pancreas, often presents with severe abdominal pain that may radiate to the back. On the other hand, heart-related pain can sometimes manifest as epigastric discomfort, particularly in women, making it crucial to consider a wide differential diagnosis when evaluating this symptom.

Diagnosis of the underlying cause of epigastric pain typically involves a thorough medical history, physical examination, and potentially imaging studies or endoscopy. Patients should be encouraged to keep a diary of their symptoms, noting any patterns related to food intake or stress, which can aid in identifying triggers. Early diagnosis and treatment are essential to managing the condition effectively and preventing complications.

Ultimately, understanding epigastric pain requires a holistic approach that considers the individual's overall health, lifestyle, and medical history. Effective communication between patients and healthcare professionals is vital to ensure accurate diagnosis and appropriate treatment. By raising awareness of this common symptom, individuals can take proactive steps towards managing their stomach health and seeking timely medical advice when necessary.

GI bleeding (haematemesis, melena)

Gastrointestinal (GI) bleeding is a serious medical condition that can manifest in various forms, including haematemesis and melena. Haematemesis refers to the vomiting of blood, which may appear bright red or have a coffee ground-like appearance. This condition often indicates bleeding from the upper GI tract, such as the oesophagus, stomach, or duodenum. It is crucial for individuals experiencing these symptoms to seek immediate medical attention, as the underlying causes can be life-threatening.

Melena, on the other hand, is characterised by black, tarry stools resulting from the digestion of blood. This indicates that the bleeding is occurring higher up in the GI tract, typically in the stomach or small intestine, where the blood has had time to be digested. Melena can be a sign of various conditions, including peptic ulcers, gastric cancer, or varices. Recognising this symptom is vital for timely diagnosis and treatment.

The causes of GI bleeding can vary widely, ranging from benign conditions to severe diseases. Common causes include peptic ulcers, gastritis, and oesophageal varices. In some cases, medications such as non-steroidal anti-inflammatory drugs (NSAIDs) can contribute to mucosal damage and bleeding. Understanding these causes is essential for both prevention and management of GI bleeding.

Diagnosis of GI bleeding typically involves a comprehensive assessment, including a medical history, physical examination, and diagnostic tests such as endoscopy or imaging studies. Endoscopy allows for direct visualisation of the GI tract, enabling healthcare providers to identify the source of bleeding and potentially treat it during the procedure. Early diagnosis is critical to improving outcomes and reducing the risk of complications.

Managing GI bleeding often requires a multidisciplinary approach, including medical treatment, lifestyle modifications, and sometimes surgical intervention. Patients are encouraged to avoid irritants such as alcohol and certain medications that can exacerbate the condition. Education about the symptoms and risks associated with GI bleeding is vital for patients, as early recognition can lead to more effective treatment and recovery.

4

Chapter 4: Gastritis and Inflammatory Conditions

Acute and chronic gastritis

Acute and chronic gastritis are two forms of inflammation affecting the stomach lining, each with distinct causes and symptoms. Acute gastritis often arises suddenly, typically triggered by factors such as excessive alcohol consumption, the use of nonsteroidal anti-inflammatory drugs (NSAIDs), or bacterial infections, particularly Helicobacter pylori. Patients may experience sharp abdominal pain, nausea, and vomiting, which can lead to dehydration and require prompt medical attention.

In contrast, chronic gastritis develops gradually and can persist for months or even years. This condition may result from prolonged exposure to irritants, such as continuous use of NSAIDs or alcohol, or can be linked to autoimmune disorders where the body's immune system mistakenly attacks the stomach lining. Symptoms of chronic gastritis may be less severe but can include chronic indigestion, a sense of fullness after meals, and a loss of appetite.

Diagnosis of both acute and chronic gastritis typically involves a combination of patient history, physical examination, and diagnostic tests, including endoscopy and biopsies. These evaluations help determine the underlying cause of the inflammation, guiding effective treatment strategies. Identifying the specific type of gastritis is crucial since management may vary significantly between acute and chronic forms.

Treatment for acute gastritis often focuses on relieving symptoms and addressing the underlying cause, which may involve discontinuing irritants such as NSAIDs or alcohol, administering antacids, or antibiotics if a bacterial infection is present. For chronic gastritis, management can include lifestyle changes, dietary adjustments, and medications to reduce stomach acid production, thereby alleviating discomfort and promoting healing of the stomach lining.

Understanding the differences between acute and chronic gastritis is essential for effective prevention and treatment. Awareness of risk factors and early symptoms can lead to timely medical intervention, reducing the risk of complications such as ulcers or gastric bleeding. Individuals experiencing persistent stomach discomfort should consult healthcare professionals for appropriate evaluation and care.

H. pylori-associated gastritis

H. pylori-associated gastritis is a condition characterised by inflammation of the stomach lining due to an infection with Helicobacter pylori, a type of bacteria. This organism is well-adapted to survive in the harsh acidic environment of the stomach and is a leading cause of various gastrointestinal disorders. The presence of H. pylori can lead to chronic gastritis, which may subsequently increase the risk of peptic ulcers and even stomach cancer if left untreated.

The symptoms of H. pylori-associated gastritis can vary among individuals, but common complaints include abdominal pain, bloating, nausea, and a feeling of fullness after eating small amounts of food. In some cases, individuals may experience no symptoms at all, which can make it difficult to diagnose the condition early. Healthcare professionals often rely on specific tests, such as breath, stool, or endoscopic biopsies, to confirm the presence of H. pylori.

Treatment typically involves a combination of antibiotics and acid-reducing medications to eradicate the bacteria and alleviate inflammation in the stomach lining. The standard treatment regimen may last from ten days to two weeks, and it is crucial for patients to complete the entire course of antibiotics to prevent the development of antibiotic resistance. Follow-up testing is often recommended to ensure that the infection has been successfully cleared.

Preventative measures are important for reducing the risk of H. pylori infection. Good hygiene practices, such as regular handwashing and consuming food and water from safe sources, can significantly lower the likelihood of transmission. Additionally, understanding the risk factors associated with H. pylori, such as living in crowded conditions or having close contact with an infected individual, can help individuals make informed decisions about their health.

In summary, H. pylori-associated gastritis is a significant health concern that can lead to more severe gastrointestinal issues if not addressed. Awareness of the symptoms, appropriate testing, and effective treatment are key to managing this condition. By adopting preventive measures, individuals can reduce their risk of infection and maintain a healthier digestive system.

Autoimmune gastritis

Autoimmune gastritis is a chronic inflammation of the stomach lining that arises when the body's immune system mistakenly attacks its own gastric cells. This condition often leads to a gradual loss of the stomach's ability to produce acid and intrinsic factor, a protein essential for vitamin B12 absorption. The causes of autoimmune gastritis are multifactorial, including genetic predisposition and environmental triggers, which can complicate its diagnosis and management.

Symptoms of autoimmune gastritis can vary widely among individuals, but common manifestations include persistent abdominal discomfort, nausea, and a feeling of fullness after eating small amounts of food. Due to the atrophy of gastric cells, patients may also experience symptoms related to vitamin B12 deficiency, such as fatigue, weakness, and neurological issues. These symptoms can significantly impact the quality of life, making early recognition and treatment crucial.

Diagnosis typically involves a combination of patient history, physical examinations, and specific tests such as endoscopy and biopsy. During an endoscopy, a doctor can visually inspect the stomach lining and obtain tissue samples to confirm the presence of inflammation and autoantibodies. Blood tests may also be conducted to evaluate vitamin B12 levels and identify autoimmune markers associated with the condition.

Treatment for autoimmune gastritis focuses on alleviating symptoms and preventing complications. This often includes vitamin B12 supplementation to address deficiencies, along with medications that help reduce stomach acid production. In some cases, lifestyle modifications, such as dietary changes and stress management, may also be recommended to support overall gastrointestinal health.

Living with autoimmune gastritis requires ongoing management and regular follow-ups with healthcare providers. Patients are encouraged to monitor their symptoms closely and seek medical advice if they experience significant changes. With proper treatment and care, individuals can lead fulfilling lives while managing this chronic condition effectively.

Radiation and caustic injury

Radiation and caustic injuries are significant concerns in the realm of stomach diseases, as they can lead to severe damage to the gastrointestinal tract. Radiation exposure may occur due to medical treatments, such as radiation therapy for cancer, or from environmental sources. The impact of radiation on the stomach can result in inflammation, ulceration, and even long-term complications if not properly managed.

Caustic injuries, on the other hand, often arise from the ingestion of harmful substances, such as strong acids or alkalis. These substances can severely damage the mucosal lining of the stomach, leading to acute pain, bleeding, and potential perforation of the stomach wall. Immediate medical intervention is crucial in these cases to mitigate the damage and prevent further complications.

The symptoms of radiation and caustic injuries can vary widely, ranging from nausea and vomiting to more severe manifestations like gastrointestinal bleeding. Patients may present with abdominal pain and discomfort, which can often lead to misdiagnosis if not carefully evaluated. Understanding the specific aetiology of these injuries is essential for appropriate treatment and management.

Treatment strategies for radiation and caustic injuries typically involve supportive care and, in some cases, surgical intervention. For radiation-induced damage, medications to alleviate symptoms and promote healing are often utilised. In contrast, caustic injuries may necessitate endoscopic procedures to remove damaged tissue or repairs to the stomach lining.

Preventive measures are vital in reducing the risk of radiation and caustic injuries. For individuals undergoing radiation therapy, proper shielding and monitoring can help minimise exposure to healthy tissues. Education on the dangers of caustic substances is equally important, particularly in households with children, to prevent accidental ingestion and ensure timely medical attention when necessary.

5

Chapter 5: Peptic Ulcer Disease (PUD)

Gastric vs. duodenal ulcers

Gastric and duodenal ulcers are both types of peptic ulcers, but they arise in different locations and have distinct characteristics. Gastric ulcers develop in the lining of the stomach, while duodenal ulcers occur in the first part of the small intestine, known as the duodenum. Understanding the differences between these two types of ulcers is essential for effective diagnosis and treatment.

The causes of gastric and duodenal ulcers often overlap, with factors such as Helicobacter pylori infection, prolonged use of non-steroidal anti-inflammatory drugs (NSAIDs), and excessive alcohol consumption playing significant roles. However, the pathophysiology can differ. Gastric ulcers tend to occur when the stomach's protective lining is compromised, often resulting from an imbalance between aggressive factors like acid and pepsin and the defensive mechanisms of the stomach lining.

In contrast, duodenal ulcers are frequently associated with increased acid secretion and are more common in younger individuals. Symptoms may vary between the two. Gastric ulcers typically cause pain shortly after eating, as the presence of food stimulates acid production, while duodenal ulcers usually result in pain that appears a few hours after a meal when the stomach is empty.

Diagnosis of both types of ulcers generally involves endoscopy and imaging studies, along with tests to detect Helicobacter pylori. Treatment strategies may include the use of proton pump inhibitors, antibiotics, and lifestyle modifications. Addressing the underlying causes is crucial to prevent recurrence and promote healing.

In summary, while gastric and duodenal ulcers share some commonalities, their differences in location, symptoms, and treatment approaches are significant. Understanding these distinctions can empower individuals to seek appropriate medical advice and make informed decisions regarding their health. Additionally, awareness of the lifestyle factors contributing to ulcer formation can aid in prevention.

Pathogenesis (H. pylori, NSAIDs, acid imbalance)

Pathogenesis in stomach diseases can often be attributed to three primary factors: Helicobacter pylori (H. pylori) infection, the use of non-steroidal anti-inflammatory drugs (NSAIDs), and acid imbalance within the stomach. H. pylori is a gram-negative bacterium that colonises the gastric mucosa, leading to chronic inflammation and ulcers. Its ability to survive in the acidic environment of the stomach is a significant factor in its pathogenicity, as it disrupts the protective mucus layer, making the gastric epithelium more susceptible to injury.

NSAIDs are commonly used medications that can exacerbate stomach issues, particularly when taken over an extended period. These drugs inhibit the production of prostaglandins, which play a crucial role in maintaining the gastric mucosal barrier. As a result, the gastrointestinal lining becomes more vulnerable to damage from gastric acid, potentially leading to gastritis or peptic ulcers. The interaction between NSAIDs and the stomach's protective mechanisms underscores the importance of cautious use in individuals with pre-existing stomach conditions.

Acid imbalance is another critical factor in the pathogenesis of stomach diseases. Conditions such as gastroesophageal reflux disease (GORD) are directly related to excessive stomach acid production or decreased oesophageal clearance. In conjunction with H. pylori infection or NSAID use, acid imbalance can accelerate the deterioration of the stomach lining, resulting in inflammation and ulcer formation. Understanding the interplay of these factors is essential for developing effective treatment strategies.

Moreover, the chronic inflammation caused by H. pylori can lead to more severe complications, including gastric cancer. The bacterium's ability to induce a persistent immune response can cause genetic alterations in gastric cells, heightening cancer risk. Regular screening for H. pylori in at-risk populations is crucial to mitigate such outcomes, as early detection can significantly alter the disease trajectory.

In summary, the pathogenesis of stomach diseases is multifaceted, involving H. pylori, NSAIDs, and acid imbalance. Awareness of these contributing factors can empower individuals to make informed decisions about their health. By understanding how these elements interact, patients and healthcare providers can work collaboratively to prevent and manage stomach-related ailments more effectively.

Diagnosis and red flags

Diagnosis of stomach diseases often begins with a thorough patient history and a physical examination. Physicians will inquire about symptoms such as abdominal pain, bloating, and changes in appetite or weight. Understanding the duration, intensity, and triggers of these symptoms can help in forming an accurate diagnosis. Additionally, patients may be asked about their dietary habits, past medical history, and any family history of gastrointestinal disorders. This comprehensive approach ensures that the underlying issues are properly identified.

Once initial information is gathered, a range of diagnostic tests may be employed. Common procedures include blood tests, endoscopies, and imaging studies such as ultrasounds or CT scans. These tests provide valuable insights into the condition of the stomach and surrounding organs. For instance, an endoscopy allows doctors to visually inspect the stomach lining and take biopsies if necessary. This thorough examination aids in distinguishing between various stomach diseases, such as gastritis, ulcers, or more serious conditions like cancer.

It is crucial to recognise red flags that may indicate a more severe problem. Symptoms such as unintentional weight loss, persistent vomiting, or blood in stools should prompt immediate medical attention. These signs can signal serious conditions that require prompt intervention. Patients should be educated about these red flags and encouraged to seek help when experiencing such symptoms, as early diagnosis often leads to better treatment outcomes.

Furthermore, lifestyle factors and risk behaviours can also play a significant role in diagnosis. Individuals with a history of excessive alcohol consumption, smoking, or prolonged use of non-steroidal anti-inflammatory drugs (NSAIDs) may be at higher risk for stomach issues. Understanding these risk factors can help healthcare providers tailor their diagnostic approach and recommend appropriate preventative measures. Awareness of personal habits and their potential impact on stomach health is an important aspect of managing and diagnosing stomach diseases.

In conclusion, the diagnosis of stomach diseases is a multifaceted process that requires careful consideration of symptoms, diagnostic testing, and recognition of red flags. By being proactive and aware of their health, individuals can play an active role in their diagnosis and treatment. The collaboration between patients and healthcare providers is essential for achieving optimal outcomes in the management of stomach diseases.

Treatment: triple/quadruple therapy, PPI, lifestyle

The treatment of stomach diseases often involves a multifaceted approach, combining medications and lifestyle changes to achieve optimal results. Triple and quadruple therapy regimens are commonly prescribed, especially for conditions like peptic ulcers and Helicobacter pylori infection. Triple therapy typically includes a proton pump inhibitor (PPI) and two antibiotics, aimed at eradicating the bacteria causing inflammation and ulceration. Quadruple therapy may add a bismuth compound, enhancing the effectiveness against stubborn infections and providing additional protective effects for the stomach lining.

Proton pump inhibitors play a crucial role in stomach disease management. These medications work by reducing gastric acid production, which aids in healing ulcers and alleviating symptoms of gastroesophageal reflux disease (GORD). By decreasing acid secretion, PPIs help to create a more favourable environment for the stomach to heal, while also providing relief from discomfort and preventing further damage to the lining.

In addition to pharmacological treatments, lifestyle modifications are essential in the management of stomach diseases. Patients are encouraged to adopt a balanced diet, avoiding foods that can exacerbate symptoms, such as spicy or acidic items. Regular physical activity and maintaining a healthy weight can also contribute significantly to improving overall gastrointestinal health. Additionally, reducing stress through mindfulness practices or relaxation techniques can further support recovery and well-being.

It is important for patients to adhere to prescribed treatment plans and maintain regular follow-ups with healthcare providers. Monitoring the effectiveness of therapy and making necessary adjustments can lead to better outcomes. Education about the condition and understanding the importance of compliance with medication and lifestyle changes can empower patients to take control of their health.

Ultimately, a comprehensive approach combining triple or quadruple therapy, PPIs, and lifestyle changes can significantly improve the quality of life for individuals suffering from stomach diseases. By addressing both the medical and lifestyle aspects, patients are more likely to experience relief from symptoms and a reduction in the recurrence of their condition. This holistic strategy is vital for long-term management and improving overall digestive health.

How NSAIDs and Aspirin Damage the Stomach

Nonsteroidal anti-inflammatory drugs (NSAIDs) and aspirin are commonly used medications for pain relief and inflammation reduction. However, their effects on the stomach can be detrimental. These drugs inhibit the production of prostaglandins, which are substances that help protect the stomach lining. Without adequate prostaglandins, the stomach becomes more susceptible to damage from its own acidic environment, leading to potential complications such as ulcers and gastritis.

The stomach lining is designed to withstand harsh acidic conditions, but the protective mechanisms can be compromised by NSAIDs and aspirin. The inhibition of prostaglandins not only reduces the protective mucus layer but also hampers the ability of the stomach to heal itself. This can result in a cycle of damage where the stomach lining becomes increasingly eroded, leading to pain, discomfort, and more severe gastrointestinal issues.

Ulcers are one of the most significant risks associated with prolonged NSAID and aspirin use. These open sores can develop on the lining of the stomach or the upper part of the small intestine, causing symptoms such as burning pain, bloating, and indigestion. In severe cases, ulcers can lead to bleeding, perforation, and even life-threatening conditions. Understanding the risks involved with these medications is crucial for anyone who relies on them for chronic pain management.

Moreover, the risk of stomach damage is heightened in certain populations, such as the elderly or those with existing gastrointestinal issues. These individuals may experience more severe side effects due to the cumulative effects of NSAIDs and aspirin on an already vulnerable stomach lining. It is essential for healthcare providers to assess the risks and benefits of these medications carefully, especially in patients with a history of gastric problems.

In conclusion, while NSAIDs and aspirin are effective for their intended purposes, their potential to damage the stomach should not be overlooked. Patients should be educated about the risks and encouraged to discuss any concerns with their physicians. Alternatives or protective strategies, such as using proton pump inhibitors, may be considered to mitigate the adverse effects on the stomach, ensuring safer management of pain and inflammation.

Other Drugs Affecting the Gastric Lining

The gastric lining is a sensitive barrier that can be affected by various drugs beyond the well-known non-steroidal anti-inflammatory drugs (NSAIDs). Many medications, including some common antibiotics and corticosteroids, have the potential to irritate the stomach lining, leading to discomfort or more severe conditions such as gastritis. Understanding the impact of these drugs is essential for individuals who rely on them for managing their health conditions while minimising risks to their digestive system.

Antibiotics, while crucial for treating infections, can disrupt the natural balance of bacteria in the stomach. This disruption can lead to an overgrowth of harmful bacteria or a decrease in protective bacterial populations, resulting in gastrointestinal issues. Some individuals may experience nausea, vomiting, or abdominal pain as side effects, highlighting the importance of monitoring the use of these medications, especially in those with a history of stomach problems.

Corticosteroids, on the other hand, are often prescribed for inflammatory conditions but can have adverse effects on the gastric lining. These drugs can increase the production of stomach acid and reduce the secretion of protective mucus, making the stomach more susceptible to irritation and ulcers. Patients using corticosteroids should be informed about these risks and may need concurrent medications to protect their gastric lining.

Other medications, including certain antidepressants and blood thinners, can also pose a risk to gastric health. Selective serotonin reuptake inhibitors (SSRIs), for instance, have been associated with gastrointestinal bleeding. Similarly, blood thinners can exacerbate any existing gastric irritation or ulcers, necessitating careful management and potential lifestyle adjustments for those who take these drugs regularly.

In conclusion, the impact of various medications on the gastric lining underscores the need for awareness and caution. Patients should engage in open discussions with their healthcare providers about the risks associated with their medications. By understanding the potential effects of these drugs, individuals can take proactive steps to protect their stomach health while effectively managing their overall medical needs.

6

Chapter 6: Functional and Motility Disorders

Functional dyspepsia

Functional dyspepsia is a common gastrointestinal disorder characterised by symptoms such as bloating, discomfort, and nausea without an identifiable organic cause. It affects a significant portion of the population and can greatly impact daily life, leading to missed work and decreased productivity. Understanding the underlying mechanisms of functional dyspepsia is crucial for both patients and healthcare providers, as it can guide effective management strategies.

The pathophysiology of functional dyspepsia is complex and multifactorial. Factors such as altered gastric motility, increased sensitivity of the gastrointestinal tract, and psychological components like stress and anxiety can all contribute to the condition. These elements often interact in a way that exacerbates symptoms, making it essential to consider a holistic approach to treatment that addresses both physical and emotional health.

Diagnosis of functional dyspepsia is primarily based on clinical history and symptom assessment, as there are no specific tests to confirm the disorder. Healthcare professionals typically rule out other potential causes of dyspepsia, such as ulcers or gastroesophageal reflux disease, before arriving at a diagnosis. This process can be frustrating for patients, who may seek answers and relief from their symptoms but find that medical evaluations yield normal results.

Management of functional dyspepsia often involves lifestyle modifications, dietary changes, and medications aimed at alleviating symptoms. Patients may benefit from keeping a food diary to identify triggers, as certain foods can worsen symptoms. Additionally, therapies such as cognitive behavioural therapy may help address underlying anxiety, leading to improved symptom control and quality of life.

In conclusion, functional dyspepsia is a prevalent condition that requires a comprehensive understanding of its causes and effects. By recognising the interplay of physiological and psychological factors, patients and healthcare providers can work together to develop effective treatment plans. Awareness and education about functional dyspepsia can significantly enhance the quality of life for those affected, making it a vital topic in the realm of stomach diseases.

Gastroparesis

Gastroparesis is a medical condition characterised by delayed gastric emptying, which means that the stomach takes longer than normal to empty its contents. This condition can lead to various symptoms, including nausea, vomiting, bloating, and abdominal pain. Individuals with gastroparesis often experience a decreased appetite and may find it challenging to eat regular meals, which can impact their nutritional status and overall health.

The exact cause of gastroparesis is not always clear, but it can be associated with several underlying health issues, such as diabetes, neurological disorders, or post-surgical complications. In diabetic patients, nerve damage caused by high blood sugar levels can disrupt the normal functioning of the stomach muscles. Furthermore, certain medications can also contribute to the slowing of gastric emptying, making it essential for individuals to consult their healthcare provider regarding their treatment options.

Diagnosis of gastroparesis typically involves a combination of medical history evaluation, physical examination, and diagnostic tests such as gastric emptying studies. During these tests, a small amount of food is ingested, and imaging is used to track how quickly it moves through the stomach. This helps healthcare professionals determine the severity of the condition and tailor a treatment plan suited to the individual's needs.

Management of gastroparesis may include dietary modifications, such as consuming smaller, more frequent meals that are low in fat and fibre, as these types of foods are easier for the stomach to process. In some cases, medications may be prescribed to stimulate gastric motility or alleviate symptoms. Additionally, in severe cases where nutritional intake is significantly compromised, enteral feeding or other interventions may be necessary to ensure adequate nutrition.

Living with gastroparesis can be challenging, as it affects daily life and the ability to enjoy food. Support from healthcare providers, nutritionists, and support groups can be invaluable for individuals coping with this condition. Understanding the intricacies of gastroparesis not only aids in managing the symptoms but also empowers patients to make informed decisions about their health and lifestyle.

Rapid gastric emptying (dumping syndrome)

Rapid gastric emptying, commonly known as dumping syndrome, occurs when food moves too quickly from the stomach into the small intestine. This condition is often observed in individuals who have undergone gastric surgery, particularly procedures that alter the stomach's size or function. The rapid transit of food can lead to a range of uncomfortable symptoms, as the body struggles to adjust to the sudden influx of nutrients into the intestines. Understanding the mechanisms behind this condition is crucial for both patients and healthcare providers to manage and alleviate its impact effectively.

Symptoms of dumping syndrome typically manifest in two phases: early and late. The early phase occurs shortly after eating and can include nausea, vomiting, abdominal cramps, and diarrhoea. These symptoms arise as the intestines react to the sudden presence of food, leading to an overwhelming demand for digestive enzymes and fluid. The late phase, which usually occurs one to three hours post-meal, is marked by symptoms such as dizziness, sweating, and increased heart rate due to a rapid drop in blood sugar levels. Recognising these symptoms is vital for timely intervention.

Dietary management plays a significant role in alleviating the symptoms of dumping syndrome. Patients are often advised to consume smaller, more frequent meals that are higher in protein and fat, which tend to slow gastric emptying. Avoiding sugary foods and beverages is also recommended, as these can exacerbate symptoms by causing a rapid influx of glucose into the bloodstream. Educating patients about appropriate food choices can empower them to take control of their condition and improve their quality of life.

In addition to dietary adjustments, other strategies may be employed to manage dumping syndrome. Some individuals may benefit from medications that slow gastric emptying or enhance nutrient absorption. In more severe cases, surgical options may be considered to correct anatomical issues contributing to the syndrome. It is essential for patients to work closely with healthcare providers to develop a personalised management plan that addresses their unique needs and circumstances.

Overall, understanding rapid gastric emptying is vital for those affected by dumping syndrome. By recognising the symptoms, implementing dietary changes, and exploring additional treatment options, individuals can significantly improve their condition. Continuous research and education on this topic are crucial for advancing treatment and enhancing the quality of life for those living with this challenging syndrome.

7

Chapter 7: Gastric Malignancies

Gastric Adenocarcinoma

Gastric adenocarcinoma is one of the most common types of stomach cancer, originating from the glandular tissues of the stomach lining. This malignancy is characterised by the uncontrolled growth of abnormal cells that can invade surrounding tissues and spread to other parts of the body. Early detection is crucial, as symptoms may often be vague and attributed to less serious gastrointestinal issues, making awareness and understanding essential for better outcomes.

The aetiology of gastric adenocarcinoma is multifactorial, with several risk factors contributing to its development. Chronic infection with Helicobacter pylori, dietary factors, smoking, and genetic predisposition are among the leading causes. Additionally, conditions such as atrophic gastritis and intestinal metaplasia increase the likelihood of developing this cancer, highlighting the importance of monitoring individuals with these conditions.

Symptoms of gastric adenocarcinoma can include persistent stomach pain, nausea, vomiting, and unexplained weight loss. As the disease progresses, patients may also experience difficulty swallowing and a feeling of fullness after eating small amounts of food. Due to the nonspecific nature of these symptoms, many patients often seek medical advice only in advanced stages, which underscores the need for public education regarding the signs and risk factors associated with this cancer.

Diagnosis typically involves a combination of endoscopy, biopsy, and imaging studies. An endoscope allows for direct visualisation of the stomach lining, while a biopsy provides tissue samples for histopathological examination. Imaging techniques, such as CT scans, help assess the extent of the disease and determine appropriate treatment options, which may include surgery, chemotherapy, and targeted therapies.

The prognosis of gastric adenocarcinoma is significantly influenced by the stage at which it is diagnosed. Early-stage detection offers better treatment outcomes, while advanced stages often correlate with a poorer prognosis. Continued research into the biology of gastric adenocarcinoma and the development of novel therapeutic approaches is vital in improving survival rates and quality of life for those affected by this disease.

Gastrointestinal Stromal Tumors (GISTs)

Gastrointestinal stromal tumours (GISTs) are a unique type of tumour that arises from the interstitial cells of Cajal in the gastrointestinal tract. These tumours can occur anywhere along the digestive system, but they are most commonly found in the stomach and small intestine. Unlike other types of cancers, GISTs are often associated with specific genetic mutations, particularly in the KIT or PDGFRA genes. Understanding these tumours is crucial for effective diagnosis and treatment, as they can behave very differently from other gastrointestinal malignancies.

The symptoms of GISTs can vary widely, with some individuals experiencing no symptoms at all, while others may present with abdominal pain, nausea, or gastrointestinal bleeding. Due to their often asymptomatic nature, GISTs can be challenging to detect in the early stages. When diagnosed, imaging techniques such as CT scans or MRI, along with endoscopic examinations, play a vital role in identifying the presence and extent of these tumours. Awareness of these symptoms is essential for timely intervention and management.

Treatment options for GISTs have evolved significantly over the past two decades. Surgical removal of the tumour is often the first line of treatment, particularly for localised cases. However, for tumours that are metastatic or unresectable, targeted therapies such as imatinib (Gleevec) have revolutionised the management of GISTs. These drugs work by inhibiting the abnormal proteins produced by the mutated genes, effectively controlling the growth of the tumours and improving patient outcomes.

Moreover, ongoing research continues to explore the biology of GISTs and the potential for new therapeutic approaches. Clinical trials are investigating novel agents and combination therapies that may further enhance treatment efficacy. The understanding of GISTs is crucial not only for developing new treatments but also for improving prognostic assessments and patient quality of life. This evolving landscape highlights the importance of continued education and awareness regarding these tumours.

In summary, GISTs represent a distinct category of gastrointestinal tumours that require a specific understanding for effective management. With advances in genetic research and treatment modalities, patients diagnosed with GISTs can achieve better outcomes than in the past. It is essential for both healthcare professionals and the public to remain informed about the characteristics and treatment options for these tumours, facilitating early diagnosis and optimal care.

Gastric Lymphomas

Gastric lymphomas are a type of cancer that originates in the stomach's lymphatic tissue. This form of lymphoma is distinct from more common gastric cancers, such as adenocarcinoma, and typically arises from the mucosa-associated lymphoid tissue (MALT). The incidence of gastric lymphomas has been increasing, highlighting the importance of understanding this disease for both patients and healthcare providers alike.

The most prevalent type of gastric lymphoma is MALT lymphoma, which is often associated with chronic inflammation, particularly due to Helicobacter pylori infection. This bacterial infection can lead to changes in the stomach lining, which may trigger the development of lymphomas. Treatment strategies often include antibiotics to eradicate H. pylori, along with other therapies tailored to the individual's specific condition.

Symptoms of gastric lymphomas can be nonspecific and may include abdominal pain, nausea, and unexplained weight loss. Due to these vague presentations, diagnosing gastric lymphomas can be challenging, and they may be mistaken for other gastrointestinal disorders. Early detection is crucial, as it can significantly improve treatment outcomes and overall prognosis.

The management of gastric lymphomas often involves a multidisciplinary approach including gastroenterologists, oncologists, and surgeons. Depending on the stage of the disease, treatment options may range from surveillance in early cases to chemotherapy and radiation for more advanced stages. Surgical intervention may also be considered in certain situations, particularly if there is a need to remove a large mass.

In conclusion, gastric lymphomas represent a unique and increasingly recognised category of stomach diseases. Understanding their aetiology, symptoms, and treatment options is essential for timely intervention and management. As research continues to evolve, it is hoped that more effective strategies will emerge to combat this complex disease and improve patient outcomes.

Screening and Surveillance

Screening and surveillance for stomach diseases play a crucial role in early detection and management. Regular screenings can help identify issues such as gastritis, ulcers, and even stomach cancer before they progress into more severe conditions. By employing various diagnostic techniques, healthcare professionals can monitor the stomach's health and ensure timely interventions when necessary.

The most common method for screening stomach diseases is through endoscopy, a procedure that allows doctors to visually examine the stomach lining. During this procedure, a thin, flexible tube with a camera is inserted through the mouth, providing real-time images of the stomach. This not only aids in diagnosis but also allows for the collection of tissue samples for further examination.

In addition to endoscopy, non-invasive tests such as breath tests and imaging studies can also be employed. Breath tests can help detect infections like Helicobacter pylori, which is a significant contributor to stomach issues. Imaging studies, including ultrasounds and CT scans, provide additional information regarding the stomach's structure and any potential abnormalities.

Surveillance is particularly important for individuals at higher risk of developing stomach diseases. Those with a family history, previous stomach issues, or specific lifestyle factors may require more frequent screenings. Regular surveillance allows for the identification of changes in the stomach that could indicate the onset of disease, thereby facilitating prompt treatment.

Ultimately, understanding the importance of screening and surveillance in stomach health empowers individuals to take proactive steps in managing their wellbeing. By being informed and engaging in regular check-ups, individuals can contribute to the early detection of potential stomach diseases, which is vital for effective treatment and improved outcomes.

8

Chapter 8: Rare and Structural Stomach Conditions

Menetrier's disease (hypertrophic gastritis)

Menetrier's disease, also known as hypertrophic gastritis, is a rare disorder characterised by the abnormal growth of the stomach lining. This condition leads to the formation of large folds in the stomach, resembling the rugae found in a healthy stomach. Although the exact cause of Menetrier's disease remains unclear, it is believed to be associated with factors such as excessive secretion of growth factors and inflammation. Patients suffering from this disease often experience symptoms like abdominal pain, nausea, and vomiting, which can significantly affect their quality of life.

Diagnosis of Menetrier's disease typically involves a combination of endoscopic examination and histological analysis of stomach tissue samples. During endoscopy, doctors can visually assess the stomach's lining and confirm the presence of the characteristic thickened folds. Biopsy samples are taken to rule out other potential conditions, such as gastric cancer, as the symptoms can often overlap. This thorough diagnostic approach is crucial for ensuring that patients receive the appropriate treatment and management of their symptoms.

Treatment options for Menetrier's disease largely focus on alleviating symptoms and addressing the underlying causes. In some cases, medications that reduce stomach acid and promote healing of the gastric lining are prescribed. For patients with more severe symptoms or complications, surgical intervention may be considered. This could involve partial or total gastrectomy, depending on the extent of the disease and the patient's overall health condition, highlighting the need for personalised treatment plans.

Living with Menetrier's disease can be challenging, as the condition may lead to nutritional deficiencies due to malabsorption of nutrients. Patients are encouraged to maintain a balanced diet and may benefit from working with a dietitian to ensure they are receiving adequate nutrition. Regular follow-up appointments with healthcare providers are also essential to monitor the disease's progression and adjust treatment plans as necessary, ensuring that patients can manage their symptoms effectively.

Research into Menetrier's disease is ongoing, with studies focusing on understanding its pathophysiology and the potential role of specific growth factors. As a rare disorder, greater awareness and understanding of Menetrier's disease among healthcare professionals and the public are vital for improving diagnosis and treatment outcomes. Enhanced knowledge can lead to better support for those affected, thereby fostering a more informed approach to managing this complex gastrointestinal condition.

Gastric polyps

Gastric polyps are abnormal growths that form on the lining of the stomach. They can vary in size and number, and while many gastric polyps are benign, some have the potential to develop into cancer. Understanding the nature of these polyps is crucial for early detection and treatment, as they may not always present noticeable symptoms. Regular medical check-ups and endoscopic examinations can help in identifying these growths before they lead to more serious conditions.

There are several types of gastric polyps, including fundic gland polyps, adenomatous polyps, and hyperplastic polyps. Fundic gland polyps are often associated with prolonged use of proton pump inhibitors and are generally considered benign. In contrast, adenomatous polyps carry a higher risk of malignancy, making them a cause for concern. Hyperplastic polyps, on the other hand, are usually non-cancerous and often arise in response to inflammation in the stomach lining.

The symptoms of gastric polyps can be quite subtle, and many individuals may remain asymptomatic. When symptoms do occur, they may include abdominal pain, nausea, vomiting, or gastrointestinal bleeding. These symptoms can often be mistaken for other stomach-related issues, making it essential for individuals to seek medical advice if they experience persistent discomfort. Early diagnosis and monitoring of gastric polyps can significantly improve outcomes and reduce the risk of developing stomach cancer.

Diagnosis of gastric polyps typically involves imaging techniques such as endoscopy, which allows for direct visualisation of the stomach lining. During an endoscopy, doctors may also perform a biopsy to determine the nature of the polyp. This process helps in identifying whether the polyp is benign or malignant, guiding the appropriate treatment plan. Depending on the findings, treatment options may range from regular surveillance to surgical removal of the polyp.

In conclusion, while gastric polyps may not always pose a significant health threat, awareness and understanding of their existence are vital. Regular check-ups and a proactive approach to stomach health can lead to early detection and effective management of any potential complications. By educating oneself about gastric polyps, individuals can take informed steps towards maintaining their digestive health and preventing more severe stomach diseases.

Bezoars

Bezoars are unusual formations that can occur in the gastrointestinal tract, often resulting from the accumulation of indigestible materials. These masses can vary in size and composition, and their presence can lead to various digestive issues. While many people may not have heard of bezoars, they can be crucial in understanding certain stomach diseases and their symptoms. Bezoars can arise from a variety of sources, including hair, vegetable fibers, and medications, making awareness of this phenomenon essential for both patients and healthcare professionals.

The formation of a bezoar typically begins when substances that are difficult to digest accumulate in the stomach or intestines. Over time, these materials can clump together, leading to a hard, stone-like mass. There are different types of bezoars, including trichobezoars, which are formed from hair, and phytobezoars, resulting from plant material. Understanding the type of bezoar is critical for determining the appropriate treatment and management strategies for affected individuals.

Symptoms associated with bezoars can vary significantly depending on their location and size. Common signs may include abdominal pain, nausea, vomiting, and changes in bowel habits. In some cases, larger bezoars may obstruct the gastrointestinal tract, leading to more severe complications that require immediate medical intervention. Therefore, recognising the symptoms early on can help in managing the condition effectively.

Diagnosis of bezoars often involves imaging techniques such as X-rays, CT scans, or ultrasounds, which can reveal the presence of these masses within the digestive system. In addition to imaging, a thorough patient history is essential to identify potential risk factors, such as previous surgeries or dietary habits that may contribute to bezoar formation. Understanding these aspects is crucial for devising preventive measures and treatment plans.

Treatment of bezoars may vary based on their size and composition. In some instances, dietary changes or medication may be sufficient to dissolve smaller bezoars. However, larger or more complicated cases might necessitate endoscopic removal or even surgical intervention. Awareness and understanding of bezoars are vital for both patients and healthcare providers, as timely intervention can prevent serious complications and improve overall digestive health.

Gastric volvulus

Gastric volvulus is a potentially life-threatening condition that occurs when the stomach twists on itself, leading to an obstruction of the digestive tract. This abnormal twisting can disrupt blood flow to the stomach, causing severe pain and a variety of gastrointestinal symptoms. Individuals experiencing gastric volvulus may present with symptoms such as abdominal distension, nausea, vomiting, and difficulty swallowing. Immediate medical attention is crucial to prevent complications, including necrosis of the stomach tissue due to compromised blood supply.

There are two primary types of gastric volvulus: organoaxial and mesenteroaxial. Organoaxial volvulus involves the stomach twisting along its long axis, while mesenteroaxial volvulus involves a twist along its short axis. The underlying causes of this condition can vary, ranging from anatomical abnormalities to prior surgical interventions that may have altered the normal structure of the stomach. Understanding these distinctions is important for accurate diagnosis and treatment planning.

Diagnosis of gastric volvulus typically involves imaging studies such as X-rays, CT scans, or endoscopy, which help to visualise the stomach's position and identify any obstructions. These diagnostic tools are vital for confirming the diagnosis and determining the best course of action. In some cases, a barium swallow test may also be utilised to observe the movement of barium through the digestive tract, providing further insight into the condition.

Treatment for gastric volvulus often requires surgical intervention to untwist the stomach and restore its normal position. In some cases, a procedure called gastropexy may be performed to secure the stomach in place and prevent future episodes. Post-operative care is essential to monitor for any complications and ensure proper recovery. Patients may also receive dietary recommendations to aid in their healing process and reduce the risk of recurrence.

Gastric volvulus is a rare but serious condition that highlights the importance of understanding stomach diseases. Awareness of the symptoms and timely medical intervention can significantly impact patient outcomes. As research continues, further insights into the causes and management of gastric volvulus may enhance our ability to treat and prevent this challenging condition effectively.

Congenital conditions

Congenital conditions affecting the stomach can significantly impact an individual's health from an early age. One such condition is pyloric stenosis, which is characterised by the narrowing of the pylorus, the opening from the stomach into the small intestine. This condition often presents in infants, typically between three and twelve weeks old, and can lead to severe vomiting and dehydration if not treated promptly. Understanding pyloric stenosis is essential for parents and caregivers to ensure timely diagnosis and intervention.

The symptoms of pyloric stenosis may include persistent vomiting, often described as projectile, as well as a constant feeling of hunger. Infants may appear to be dehydrated, which can be identified by fewer wet nappies, dry mouth, and lethargy. As the condition progresses, the infant may also develop a notable abdominal mass, often referred to as a "olive-like" structure, which can be felt during a physical examination. Recognising these signs early is crucial as they can help differentiate pyloric stenosis from other gastrointestinal issues.

Diagnosis of pyloric stenosis typically involves a combination of physical examination and imaging tests, such as an abdominal ultrasound. The ultrasound is particularly effective in visualising the narrowed pylorus and confirming the diagnosis. Once diagnosed, the primary treatment for pyloric stenosis is surgical intervention, known as a pyloromyotomy, which involves cutting the muscle to relieve the obstruction. This procedure is usually performed laparoscopically, resulting in less pain and quicker recovery for the infant.

Post-surgery, most infants can resume normal feeding within a few hours, and the prognosis is generally excellent. Most children recover fully and grow without any long-term complications related to the condition. However, it's important for parents to monitor their child's feeding and behaviour during recovery, as some may experience temporary digestive issues. Regular follow-up with a healthcare provider ensures that the infant is thriving and developing appropriately.

In conclusion, congenital conditions like pyloric stenosis highlight the importance of awareness and understanding among caregivers. Early recognition of symptoms and prompt medical intervention can lead to successful outcomes and healthy growth for affected infants. By familiarising themselves with the signs and treatment options, parents can play a crucial role in managing their child's health effectively.

9

Chapter 9: Bariatric Surgery and the Stomach

Overview and Indications

Stomach diseases encompass a wide range of conditions that affect the structure and function of the stomach. These diseases can vary significantly in their aetiologies, symptoms, and potential complications. Understanding the basics of stomach diseases is crucial for early diagnosis and effective management. This chapter aims to provide an overview of various stomach diseases and their indications, helping readers to recognise potential issues and seek appropriate medical advice.

Among the most common stomach diseases are gastritis, peptic ulcer disease, and gastroesophageal reflux disease (GORD). Gastritis refers to the inflammation of the stomach lining, which can be caused by factors such as infection, excessive alcohol consumption, or prolonged use of certain medications. Peptic ulcers are sores that develop on the stomach lining or the upper part of the small intestine, typically due to the bacteria Helicobacter pylori or the use of nonsteroidal anti-inflammatory drugs (NSAIDs). GORD involves the backflow of stomach acid into the oesophagus, leading to symptoms such as heartburn and regurgitation.

Recognising the symptoms associated with stomach diseases is essential for timely intervention. Common symptoms may include abdominal pain, bloating, nausea, vomiting, and changes in appetite. These symptoms can range from mild to severe, and their duration may vary. In some cases, individuals may experience alarming signs such as persistent vomiting, blood in the stool, or significant weight loss, which warrant immediate medical attention. Understanding these indications can empower individuals to take proactive steps in managing their health.

Diagnosis of stomach diseases often involves a combination of patient history, physical examinations, and diagnostic tests. Healthcare professionals may recommend endoscopy, imaging studies, or laboratory tests to confirm the presence of a specific condition. Each diagnostic tool plays a vital role in determining the underlying cause of symptoms and guides appropriate treatment strategies. Early and accurate diagnosis is paramount to prevent complications and improve patient outcomes.

In conclusion, a comprehensive understanding of stomach diseases and their indications is vital for both patients and healthcare providers. Awareness of symptoms, risk factors, and available diagnostic methods can facilitate early intervention and effective management. By fostering a greater understanding of these conditions, individuals can better navigate their health journeys and collaborate with healthcare professionals to ensure optimal care.

Types of Bariatric Surgery

Bariatric surgery encompasses various surgical procedures aimed at aiding weight loss for individuals suffering from obesity. These surgeries work by modifying the digestive system to limit food intake, reduce nutrient absorption, or both. The most common types of bariatric surgery include gastric bypass, sleeve gastrectomy, and adjustable gastric banding, each with its unique mechanisms and benefits. Understanding these different types is essential for patients considering this life-altering option.

Gastric bypass surgery involves creating a small pouch at the top of the stomach, which is then connected directly to the small intestine. This procedure significantly reduces the amount of food that can be consumed and alters the digestive process, leading to reduced calorie and nutrient intake. Gastric bypass is often recommended for patients with a higher body mass index (BMI) and those suffering from obesity-related health issues, such as diabetes or hypertension.

Sleeve gastrectomy is another prevalent type of bariatric surgery, which involves removing a large portion of the stomach, leaving a smaller, sleeve-shaped stomach. This surgery not only limits food intake but also affects hormones that regulate appetite, resulting in reduced hunger and food cravings. Sleeve gastrectomy has gained popularity due to its effectiveness and the relatively straightforward nature of the procedure compared to other types of bariatric surgeries.

Adjustable gastric banding, commonly known as lap band surgery, involves placing an adjustable band around the upper part of the stomach. This band creates a small pouch that restricts food intake and can be adjusted over time, allowing for personalised weight loss management. While it is a less invasive option, the success rate may vary, and it requires ongoing medical supervision to ensure effectiveness.

In conclusion, understanding the various types of bariatric surgery is crucial for anyone considering this option to tackle obesity. Each type has distinct advantages and risks, and the choice of procedure should be made in consultation with a qualified healthcare professional. Patients should consider their individual health needs and weight loss goals when exploring these surgical options.

How They Work: Hormonal and Mechanical Effects

The functioning of the stomach involves a complex interplay of hormonal and mechanical effects that are crucial for digestion. Hormones such as gastrin, secretin, and cholecystokinin play significant roles in regulating stomach function, influencing the secretion of gastric juices and the movement of food through the digestive tract. Gastrin, for instance, stimulates the production of gastric acid, essential for breaking down food, while secretin and cholecystokinin help regulate the release of digestive enzymes from the pancreas and bile from the gallbladder.

Mechanical effects also contribute to the stomach's function, primarily through the muscular contractions known as peristalsis. These contractions help mix food with gastric juices, creating a semi-liquid substance called chyme. As food enters the stomach, the muscular walls expand and contract rhythmically, facilitating the mixing process and ensuring that the food is adequately broken down before moving into the small intestine. This mechanical action is vital for effective digestion and nutrient absorption.

The hormonal signals governing stomach function are intricately linked to the mechanical processes. For example, when food enters the stomach, it triggers the release of gastrin, which in turn stimulates gastric motility. This relationship illustrates how hormonal communication can enhance mechanical actions, ensuring that the digestive system operates efficiently. Disruptions in either hormonal balance or mechanical function can lead to various stomach diseases, highlighting the importance of both aspects in maintaining digestive health.

Moreover, the interplay between hormones and mechanical effects is not static; it can be influenced by various factors, including stress, diet, and overall health. For instance, stress can alter hormone levels, which may impact motility and contribute to conditions such as gastritis or gastroesophageal reflux disease (GORD). Understanding these interactions is essential for developing effective treatments and management strategies for stomach diseases, emphasising the need for a holistic approach to digestive health.

In conclusion, the harmonious functioning of hormonal and mechanical effects within the stomach is fundamental to the digestive process. By appreciating how these systems work together, individuals can gain insights into the complexities of stomach diseases and the importance of maintaining a balanced digestive environment. This understanding can empower patients and healthcare providers alike to make informed decisions regarding diet, lifestyle, and medical interventions, ultimately promoting better digestive health.

Long-Term Effects and Nutritional Considerations

Long-term effects of stomach diseases can significantly impact an individual's overall health and quality of life. Chronic conditions such as gastritis or peptic ulcers may lead to persistent discomfort and complications that extend beyond the digestive system. For instance, the malabsorption of nutrients can occur due to prolonged inflammation, which may result in deficiencies that affect various bodily functions. Therefore, understanding these potential long-term effects is crucial for effective management and treatment.

Nutritional considerations are paramount for individuals suffering from stomach diseases. A balanced diet tailored to accommodate specific digestive issues can help alleviate symptoms and promote healing. Foods that are easy to digest, such as bananas, rice, and applesauce, are often recommended during flare-ups. Conversely, spicy, fatty, or highly acidic foods may need to be avoided to prevent irritation and exacerbation of symptoms.

Moreover, hydration plays a vital role in managing stomach diseases. Adequate fluid intake is essential to facilitate digestion and nutrient absorption. Dehydration can worsen the condition, leading to further complications. Individuals should aim to drink water regularly and consider electrolyte-rich fluids if they experience vomiting or diarrhoea, which can deplete essential minerals and fluids from the body.

Another important aspect of nutritional management is the timing and frequency of meals. Smaller, more frequent meals can help reduce the burden on the digestive system compared to larger meals. This approach allows for better digestion and can help prevent episodes of discomfort. Additionally, incorporating probiotics into the diet may support gut health by restoring the balance of beneficial bacteria, which can be disrupted by stomach diseases.

Lastly, it is advisable for individuals with stomach diseases to consult healthcare professionals for personalised dietary recommendations. Each person's condition and nutritional needs can vary greatly, making tailored advice essential. Regular monitoring and adjustments to one's diet can lead to improved health outcomes and a better quality of life for those navigating the challenges of stomach diseases.

10

Chapter 10: Diagnostic Tools in Gastric Disease

Endoscopy (EGD)

Endoscopy, specifically oesophagogastroduodenoscopy (EGD), is a pivotal diagnostic procedure used to visualise the upper gastrointestinal (GI) tract. This procedure involves the insertion of a flexible tube equipped with a camera into the mouth, allowing healthcare professionals to examine the oesophagus, stomach, and duodenum. EGD is particularly beneficial in diagnosing conditions such as ulcers, tumours, and inflammation, providing direct visual access to areas that are otherwise difficult to assess.

During an EGD, patients are typically sedated to ensure comfort throughout the procedure. A local anaesthetic may also be applied to the throat to minimise gag reflex. The endoscope transmits images to a monitor, enabling the physician to identify any abnormalities. This direct visualisation is invaluable, as it allows for immediate assessment and potential biopsies if suspicious tissues are found.

The procedure is often recommended for individuals experiencing chronic gastrointestinal symptoms such as persistent heartburn, unexplained weight loss, or difficulty swallowing. Early diagnosis through EGD can lead to more effective treatment plans, significantly improving patient outcomes. It is essential for patients to discuss any concerns with their healthcare provider prior to the procedure, ensuring they are well-informed about what to expect.

Post-procedure, patients may experience a sore throat or bloating, but these symptoms typically resolve quickly. Most individuals can resume normal activities within a day, although it is advisable to avoid driving or operating heavy machinery for the remainder of the day due to the sedative effects. Follow-up appointments may be scheduled to discuss the findings and any necessary next steps in their treatment.

In conclusion, EGD is an essential tool in the field of gastroenterology, offering a minimally invasive means to diagnose and manage stomach diseases. By understanding the procedure and its benefits, patients can actively participate in their healthcare decisions. Awareness of the signs that warrant an EGD can lead to timely interventions, ultimately enhancing gastrointestinal health and overall well-being.

Urea breath test

The urea breath test is a non-invasive diagnostic procedure used primarily to detect the presence of Helicobacter pylori, a bacterium that is often implicated in various stomach diseases, including peptic ulcers and gastritis. This test measures the amount of carbon dioxide in the breath after the patient ingests a urea solution labelled with a specific isotope. If H. pylori is present in the stomach, it will metabolise the urea, producing carbon dioxide that is then absorbed into the bloodstream and eventually exhaled in the breath.

Before undergoing the test, patients are usually advised to avoid certain medications, particularly antibiotics and proton pump inhibitors, for a specified period. This is crucial as these substances can interfere with the accuracy of the test results. Additionally, fasting for a few hours prior to the test may also be required to ensure optimal conditions for measurement. The procedure itself is quick and generally well-tolerated, making it a preferred choice for both clinicians and patients.

Once the breath samples are collected, they are analysed in a laboratory to determine the presence of the labelled carbon dioxide. A positive result indicates an active H. pylori infection, while a negative result suggests that the bacterium is absent or that it is not currently causing an infection. This test not only aids in diagnosis but also helps in monitoring the effectiveness of treatment for those already diagnosed with H. pylori-related conditions.

The advantages of the urea breath test include its simplicity, accuracy, and minimal discomfort for patients. Unlike endoscopic procedures, which are invasive and require sedation, the urea breath test can be performed in a standard outpatient setting. This contributes to a more streamlined approach to diagnosing stomach diseases, allowing for quicker treatment decisions.

In conclusion, the urea breath test serves as a vital tool in the assessment of stomach health. Its ability to provide reliable information on the presence of H. pylori makes it an essential component in the management of stomach diseases. As awareness of gastrointestinal health continues to grow, understanding the role of this test will empower patients and healthcare providers alike to make informed decisions about treatment options.

H. pylori stool antigen

H. pylori, short for Helicobacter pylori, is a type of bacteria that can infect the stomach lining, leading to various gastrointestinal issues. The presence of H. pylori is a significant contributor to stomach ulcers and chronic gastritis. To diagnose this infection, one of the most effective methods employed is the stool antigen test. This non-invasive procedure detects specific antigens produced by the bacteria in a stool sample, providing a clear indication of an active infection.

The stool antigen test is preferred for its convenience and accuracy. Unlike endoscopic procedures, which require sedation and carry more risks, the stool test can be performed in a doctor's office or even at home, making it accessible to a wider population. The results from the test can help guide treatment options, allowing healthcare providers to prescribe appropriate antibiotics or proton pump inhibitors to eradicate the infection and alleviate symptoms.

Understanding the mechanism of the stool antigen test is crucial for recognising its importance in diagnosing H. pylori infections. The test works by identifying proteins that the bacteria shed into the stool, which are specific to H. pylori. A positive result indicates that the bacteria are present and actively infecting the stomach lining. It is essential to follow up on positive test results with further evaluation to determine the extent of the infection and any potential complications.

In addition to its diagnostic utility, the stool antigen test plays a vital role in monitoring treatment efficacy. After a course of antibiotics, a follow-up stool test can confirm whether the infection has been successfully eradicated. This step is critical in preventing the recurrence of ulcers and other related stomach diseases, ensuring that patients receive effective and timely care.

In conclusion, the H. pylori stool antigen test is a key tool in the diagnosis and management of stomach diseases caused by Helicobacter pylori. Its non-invasive nature, combined with its accuracy, makes it a preferred choice for clinicians and patients alike. Understanding this test empowers individuals to take proactive steps towards their gastrointestinal health, fostering better outcomes in the fight against stomach-related ailments.

Gastric pH monitoring

Gastric pH monitoring is a crucial aspect of understanding stomach diseases, as it provides insight into the acidity levels within the stomach. The pH level in the gastric environment plays a significant role in digestion and can indicate various health issues. By measuring the gastric pH, healthcare professionals can assess how well the stomach is functioning and identify any abnormalities that may contribute to discomfort or disease.

One common method for monitoring gastric pH is through the use of a pH probe, which is inserted into the stomach via the nasal passage. This probe continuously measures the acidity levels over a specified period, allowing for an accurate assessment of gastric function. Patients may be advised to keep a diary of their symptoms during the monitoring period, which can help correlate pH levels with episodes of discomfort or other gastrointestinal issues.

Abnormal gastric pH levels can indicate conditions such as gastroesophageal reflux disease (GORD) or peptic ulcers. In patients with GORD, for example, the pH may be higher than normal due to the frequent backflow of stomach acid into the oesophagus. Conversely, low pH levels can suggest an overproduction of acid, which can lead to irritation of the stomach lining and the development of ulcers.

The results of gastric pH monitoring can guide treatment decisions and lifestyle modifications. For instance, if high acidity is detected, a physician may recommend dietary changes or prescribe medications that reduce acid production. Understanding the pH levels can empower patients to make informed choices about their diets and lifestyle, ultimately leading to better management of their stomach health.

In conclusion, gastric pH monitoring is an essential tool for diagnosing and managing stomach diseases. By providing valuable information about the acidity levels in the stomach, it allows healthcare providers to tailor treatment plans to individual needs. This proactive approach can enhance patient outcomes and contribute to a greater understanding of the complexities of stomach health.

Imaging (CT, barium meal)

Imaging techniques play a vital role in diagnosing and understanding stomach diseases. Among these, Computed Tomography (CT) scans and barium meal studies are two commonly used methods. CT scans provide detailed cross-sectional images of the stomach and surrounding organs, allowing healthcare professionals to identify abnormalities such as tumours, inflammation, or structural issues. This non-invasive technique is particularly useful for assessing the extent of diseases and planning appropriate treatments.

Barium meal studies, on the other hand, involve the ingestion of a barium-based contrast material, which helps to enhance the visibility of the stomach lining during X-ray imaging. This method is particularly effective in diagnosing conditions like ulcers, blockages, and gastroesophageal reflux disease (GORD). The barium coats the stomach and highlights any irregularities, making it easier for doctors to evaluate the organ's function and structure.

Both imaging techniques offer unique advantages and can often be complementary in clinical practice. While CT scans provide a comprehensive view of the abdominal area, barium meal studies focus specifically on the stomach's interior. This combination can lead to more accurate diagnoses and better-informed treatment decisions. Furthermore, advancements in imaging technology continue to improve the resolution and speed of these procedures, enhancing their effectiveness.

It is important for patients to understand what to expect during these imaging processes. For a CT scan, patients may need to fast for a few hours beforehand, and they might receive a contrast dye to improve the visibility of the stomach. In contrast, a barium meal study requires the patient to drink a barium solution, which can be a bit unpleasant but is generally safe. Both procedures are typically quick, with minimal discomfort involved.

In conclusion, imaging techniques such as CT scans and barium meal studies are essential tools in the diagnosis of stomach diseases. They provide valuable insights that guide treatment and management strategies. Understanding these imaging methods can help patients feel more informed and at ease when undergoing these important diagnostic procedures.

Gastric emptying studies

Gastric emptying studies are vital diagnostic tools used to assess the rate at which food leaves the stomach and enters the small intestine. These studies can help identify conditions such as gastroparesis, where the stomach takes too long to empty its contents, leading to symptoms like nausea, vomiting, and bloating. By understanding gastric emptying, healthcare professionals can better diagnose and treat various stomach diseases that affect digestion.

11

Chapter 11: Medications for Stomach Disorders

Proton Pump Inhibitors (PPI)

Proton Pump Inhibitors (PPIs) are a class of medications widely used to treat various stomach-related conditions, particularly those involving excessive stomach acid production. They work by blocking the proton pump in the stomach lining, which is responsible for secreting hydrochloric acid. This action effectively reduces the acidity in the stomach, providing relief from symptoms of conditions such as gastroesophageal reflux disease (GORD), peptic ulcers, and Zollinger-Ellison syndrome.

The use of PPIs has significantly transformed the management of acid-related disorders. By lowering acid levels, these medications not only alleviate discomfort but also promote healing of the oesophagus and stomach lining. Popular PPIs include omeprazole, esomeprazole, and lansoprazole, which are often available both over-the-counter and by prescription. Their effectiveness has made them a go-to option for many healthcare providers treating patients with acid-related ailments.

Despite their benefits, the long-term use of PPIs has raised concerns among healthcare professionals and patients alike. Research has indicated that prolonged use may be associated with several potential side effects, including an increased risk of fractures, kidney disease, and gastrointestinal infections. It is crucial for patients to discuss the duration and necessity of PPI therapy with their healthcare provider to mitigate these risks while still managing their symptoms effectively.

Moreover, the mechanism of action of PPIs highlights their importance in modern medicine. By inhibiting the final step of acid production, these medications provide a powerful tool in controlling gastric acidity. This is particularly important for patients suffering from conditions where acid exposure can lead to significant complications, such as Barrett's oesophagus, a precursor to oesophageal cancer. Therefore, understanding how PPIs function can empower patients to make informed decisions regarding their treatment options.

In summary, Proton Pump Inhibitors represent a critical advancement in the treatment of stomach diseases tied to acid production. While they offer considerable benefits in symptom relief and healing, awareness of their potential risks is essential. Patients must engage in open dialogue with their healthcare providers to ensure that they receive the most appropriate and safe care for their individual needs. Education about PPIs and their role in managing stomach diseases contributes to better health outcomes and patient satisfaction.

H2 Receptor Antagonists

H2 receptor antagonists, also known as H2 blockers, play a significant role in the management of various stomach diseases, particularly those related to excessive stomach acid production. These medications work by inhibiting the action of histamine on H2 receptors located in the gastric parietal cells, which are responsible for acid secretion. By blocking these receptors, H2 antagonists effectively reduce the volume of gastric acid released into the stomach, providing relief from symptoms associated with conditions such as gastroesophageal reflux disease (GORD) and peptic ulcers.

The introduction of H2 receptor antagonists in the late 20th century revolutionised the treatment of acid-related disorders. Commonly used drugs in this category include ranitidine, famotidine, and cimetidine. Each of these medications varies slightly in potency and duration of action, but they all serve the same fundamental purpose: to alleviate discomfort caused by excessive acidity. Their ability to provide symptomatic relief has made them a staple in both over-the-counter and prescription medications.

H2 antagonists are generally well-tolerated, with a relatively low incidence of side effects. Common side effects may include headaches, dizziness, and gastrointestinal disturbances. However, serious adverse effects are rare, making them a preferred choice for many patients. It is important, though, for individuals to consult healthcare professionals before starting any new medication, as potential drug interactions and contraindications must be considered, especially in those with pre-existing health conditions.

In addition to their role in treating established conditions, H2 receptor antagonists are also used for prophylactic measures. For example, they may be prescribed to individuals at risk of developing stress-related mucosal disease, particularly in hospital settings. They help in preventing ulcers in patients who are critically ill or undergoing major surgery, thereby ensuring better gastrointestinal health during recovery periods.

While H2 receptor antagonists are effective, they are not without limitations. Long-term use has been associated with potential rebound acid hypersecretion and changes in gut flora. As such, healthcare providers often recommend lifestyle modifications and dietary changes alongside pharmacological treatments for optimal management of stomach diseases. Understanding these factors can empower patients to make informed decisions about their treatment options and overall health.

Prokinetics (domperidone, metoclopramide)

Prokinetics are a class of medications that enhance gastrointestinal motility, making them particularly useful in treating various stomach ailments. Two of the most commonly prescribed prokinetics are domperidone and metoclopramide. These medications work by increasing the movement of food through the stomach and intestines, which can alleviate symptoms such as nausea, vomiting, and bloating. Understanding how these drugs function can provide insight into their effectiveness and potential side effects.

Domperidone primarily acts on the peripheral dopamine receptors in the gastrointestinal tract. By blocking these receptors, domperidone increases the motility of the stomach and improves gastric emptying. This medication is often prescribed for patients experiencing nausea and vomiting due to conditions such as gastroparesis or as a side effect of certain medications. Its efficacy in managing symptoms makes it a valuable option in the treatment of various stomach diseases.

Metoclopramide, on the other hand, works by blocking dopamine receptors in both the central and peripheral nervous systems. This dual action not only enhances gastrointestinal motility but also has antiemetic properties, making it effective for patients suffering from chemotherapy-induced nausea or post-operative nausea. However, metoclopramide is associated with a higher incidence of side effects, particularly neurological ones, which necessitates careful monitoring during treatment.

Both medications can be beneficial, but they are not without risks. Side effects for domperidone may include dry mouth, dizziness, and, in rare cases, cardiac complications. Metoclopramide's potential side effects include fatigue, drowsiness, and the risk of tardive dyskinesia, a serious movement disorder. It is crucial for healthcare providers to evaluate the benefits against the risks when prescribing these medications, ensuring they are used appropriately.

In conclusion, prokinetics like domperidone and metoclopramide offer significant therapeutic benefits for patients suffering from various gastrointestinal disorders. Their ability to enhance motility and alleviate symptoms is essential in managing stomach diseases effectively. However, understanding the potential side effects and risks associated with these medications is vital for ensuring patient safety and optimal treatment outcomes.

Sucralfate, antacids, mucosal protectants

Sucralfate, a medication widely used in the treatment of stomach diseases, functions primarily as a mucosal protectant. It works by forming a protective barrier over ulcers and inflamed areas in the stomach lining, thereby promoting healing and reducing pain. This mechanism is particularly beneficial for individuals suffering from peptic ulcers, as it provides a physical shield against stomach acid and digestive enzymes.

Antacids, another vital component in managing stomach ailments, function by neutralising stomach acid. These over-the-counter medications provide rapid relief from symptoms such as heartburn and indigestion. By increasing the pH level in the stomach, antacids can alleviate discomfort and create a more favourable environment for healing.

Mucosal protectants, including sucralfate, play a crucial role in safeguarding the stomach's lining from irritants. They not only form a barrier but also stimulate the production of mucus and bicarbonate, which are essential for maintaining the integrity of the gastric mucosa. This dual action helps to prevent further damage and encourages the body's natural healing processes.

The combination of sucralfate and antacids can be particularly effective in treating various stomach conditions. While antacids provide immediate relief from acid-related symptoms, sucralfate offers a longer-term solution by promoting healing of the gastric lining. This synergy makes it a popular choice among healthcare providers for managing chronic stomach issues.

In conclusion, understanding the roles of sucralfate, antacids, and mucosal protectants is essential for anyone dealing with stomach diseases. Recognising how these medications work can empower patients to make informed decisions about their treatment options. By effectively managing symptoms and promoting healing, these medications contribute significantly to improving the quality of life for individuals with stomach disorders.

Antibiotics for H. pylori

Helicobacter pylori, often abbreviated as H. pylori, is a type of bacteria that can infect the stomach lining. This infection is a significant contributor to various stomach diseases, including gastritis, peptic ulcers, and even stomach cancer. The treatment of H. pylori typically involves a specific regimen of antibiotics, which are crucial in eradicating the bacteria from the gastrointestinal tract. Understanding the role of antibiotics in this context is essential for anyone interested in stomach health.

Antibiotics work by targeting and killing the bacteria, thereby alleviating the symptoms associated with H. pylori infection. The most commonly used antibiotics include amoxicillin, clarithromycin, and metronidazole. These medications are often prescribed in combination with proton pump inhibitors, which help reduce stomach acid and enhance the effectiveness of the antibiotics. This combination therapy is known as triple therapy and is the standard approach for treating H. pylori infections.

The duration of antibiotic treatment for H. pylori usually lasts between 10 to 14 days. It is essential for patients to complete the full course of antibiotics to ensure the complete eradication of the bacteria. Failure to do so may result in antibiotic resistance, making future treatments less effective. Therefore, adherence to the prescribed treatment regimen is critical for successful outcomes.

While antibiotics are effective, they can also lead to side effects, such as nausea, diarrhoea, and abdominal pain. Patients should be informed about these potential side effects and encouraged to report any severe reactions to their healthcare provider. It is also vital to discuss any other medications or health conditions, as these can influence the choice of antibiotics and overall treatment plan.

In conclusion, the use of antibiotics for treating H. pylori is a vital component in the management of stomach diseases. Their role in eradicating the bacteria can significantly improve a patient's quality of life and reduce the risk of severe complications. Ongoing research continues to explore more effective treatment regimens, especially in the face of growing antibiotic resistance, ensuring that patients receive the best possible care for their stomach health.

12

Chapter 12: Lifestyle, Diet, and Mental Health

Role of diet in symptom management

Diet plays a crucial role in the management of stomach diseases, influencing both the severity of symptoms and overall health. A balanced diet can help alleviate discomfort caused by various conditions such as gastritis, ulcers, and reflux. Understanding the specific dietary needs and restrictions associated with these diseases is essential for effective symptom management.

Certain foods can exacerbate symptoms, while others can provide relief. For instance, spicy foods, caffeine, and alcohol are often triggers for individuals suffering from acid reflux or gastritis. Conversely, a diet rich in fruits, vegetables, and whole grains can promote healing and reduce inflammation in the stomach lining.

Hydration is another critical aspect of diet that should not be overlooked. Drinking adequate amounts of water aids digestion and helps in the absorption of nutrients. Herbal teas, such as chamomile or ginger, can also soothe the stomach and provide comfort during flare-ups.

Moreover, portion control and meal timing are essential components of managing stomach diseases. Eating smaller, more frequent meals can prevent overloading the stomach, reducing the risk of discomfort and indigestion. Listening to one's body and noticing how different foods affect symptoms is vital for tailoring a diet that works.

In conclusion, diet is a powerful tool in the management of stomach diseases. By making informed dietary choices and being mindful of food triggers, individuals can significantly improve their quality of life. Consulting with a healthcare professional or a dietitian can provide personalised guidance and support in navigating dietary changes.

Stress, anxiety, and functional symptoms

Stress and anxiety are increasingly recognised as significant contributors to various stomach diseases. These emotional states can trigger or exacerbate gastrointestinal symptoms, leading to a cycle of discomfort and distress. Individuals experiencing stress may find that their digestive systems become more sensitive, resulting in issues such as bloating, pain, or irregular bowel movements. Understanding the link between mental health and stomach function is crucial for effective management of these conditions.

The connection between the brain and the gut is often referred to as the gut-brain axis. This bi-directional communication pathway means that psychological factors can influence physical health, including gastrointestinal function. Stress hormones can alter gut motility, secretion of digestive enzymes, and the overall microbiome balance. As a result, individuals with high levels of anxiety may experience more pronounced symptoms of stomach diseases, necessitating a holistic approach to treatment.

Functional symptoms, which include discomfort without an identifiable organic cause, are particularly common in the context of stress and anxiety. Conditions such as irritable bowel syndrome (IBS) exemplify how psychological factors can manifest physically. Patients might endure significant abdominal pain or altered bowel habits without any observable abnormalities in medical tests. This highlights the need for healthcare professionals to consider both mental and physical health when diagnosing and managing stomach issues.

Moreover, the experience of living with chronic stomach conditions can itself lead to increased anxiety and stress. The unpredictability of symptoms can create a significant burden, affecting an individual's quality of life. Support from mental health professionals, alongside medical treatment, can be beneficial in breaking this cycle. Patients are encouraged to engage in stress-reducing activities such as mindfulness, meditation, or counselling to help alleviate their symptoms.

In conclusion, addressing stress and anxiety is essential for those suffering from stomach diseases. A comprehensive approach that includes psychological support, lifestyle changes, and medical treatment can lead to improved outcomes. By recognising the interplay between mental and physical health, individuals can take proactive steps towards managing their conditions more effectively, ultimately leading to a better quality of life.

The gut-brain axis and stomach

The gut-brain axis is a complex communication network linking the gastrointestinal tract and the brain, playing a crucial role in both physical and mental health. This bidirectional communication pathway allows the gut to influence brain function and vice versa, highlighting the importance of gut health in overall well-being. Understanding this connection is vital for addressing various stomach diseases and their psychological impacts, as the gut microbiota can impact mood, behaviour, and cognitive functions.

Recent research has shown that the gut microbiome, a community of microbes residing in the digestive tract, can significantly affect the gut-brain axis. These microbes produce neurotransmitters and other metabolites that can reach the brain, influencing emotions and cognitive processes. This relationship underscores the potential for dietary changes and probiotic interventions to promote mental health through the modulation of gut flora, suggesting a promising avenue for treating stomach-related disorders.

The stomach, as a key organ in the digestive system, plays a significant role in this axis. It is not only responsible for breaking down food but also releases hormones and signals that can affect the brain's functioning. For instance, stress and anxiety can lead to gastrointestinal disturbances, which in turn can exacerbate psychological conditions, creating a vicious cycle. This interplay between the stomach and the brain illustrates the need for a holistic approach to treating stomach diseases, considering both physical and mental health aspects.

Moreover, conditions such as irritable bowel syndrome (IBS) and inflammatory bowel disease (IBD) often present with psychological comorbidities, including anxiety and depression. Understanding the gut-brain axis can aid in developing comprehensive treatment strategies that address both the gastrointestinal symptoms and the mental health challenges faced by patients. This approach can lead to improved outcomes and a better quality of life for individuals suffering from these chronic conditions.

In conclusion, the gut-brain axis represents a fascinating area of study that bridges our understanding of stomach diseases and mental health. By recognising the interconnections between the gut and the brain, healthcare professionals can enhance their treatment modalities, offering more effective and personalised care for patients. Continued research in this field promises to unveil new insights into how we can better manage stomach diseases and improve overall health.

Alcohol, caffeine, and smoking effects

The consumption of alcohol, caffeine, and tobacco products can significantly impact stomach health and overall digestive function. Alcohol, while often enjoyed socially, can irritate the stomach lining, leading to inflammation and gastritis. Regular heavy drinking may exacerbate these issues, resulting in a higher risk of ulcers and long-term complications such as liver disease, which can further affect digestion.

Caffeine, found in coffee, tea, and many soft drinks, can stimulate gastric acid secretion. While moderate amounts might not pose a significant threat, excessive caffeine intake can lead to increased acid levels, which may aggravate conditions like acid reflux or gastroesophageal reflux disease (GORD). Individuals with sensitive stomachs or pre-existing conditions should monitor their caffeine consumption closely to avoid exacerbating their symptoms.

Smoking also plays a detrimental role in stomach health. The chemicals present in tobacco can weaken the lower oesophageal sphincter, increasing the likelihood of acid reflux. Furthermore, smoking is linked to a higher incidence of peptic ulcers and can hinder the healing process of existing gastrointestinal issues, making it crucial for smokers to consider the impact of their habit on their stomach health.

Combining alcohol, caffeine, and smoking may create a compounded effect that can be particularly harmful. For instance, drinking alcohol while consuming caffeine could mask the sedative effects of alcohol, leading individuals to drink more than they realise, which can increase the risk of digestive issues. Additionally, the combined irritants may overwhelm the stomach, resulting in symptoms such as heartburn, nausea, and abdominal pain.

Overall, understanding the effects of alcohol, caffeine, and smoking on stomach health is essential for anyone looking to maintain good digestive function. Making informed choices regarding these substances can help prevent complications and promote overall well-being. Individuals with existing stomach conditions, in particular, should be aware of these influences and consider reducing their intake to improve their health outcomes.

13

Chapter 13: Future Trends and Innovations

New acid blockers and mucosal protectors

Acid blockers and mucosal protectors play a crucial role in the management of stomach diseases. These medications are designed to alleviate symptoms associated with excessive stomach acid and to protect the stomach lining from damage. As medical research continues to advance, new formulations and drugs are being developed to enhance efficacy and minimise side effects. Understanding these new options is essential for anyone dealing with gastrointestinal issues.

New acid blockers, such as the latest proton pump inhibitors (PPIs), offer improved mechanisms of action that can lead to faster relief from acid-related disorders. These medications work by effectively reducing the production of stomach acid, thereby providing patients with a much-needed reprieve from conditions like gastroesophageal reflux disease (GORD) and peptic ulcers. The introduction of long-acting formulations also means that patients can experience prolonged symptom relief with fewer daily doses.

In addition to acid blockers, mucosal protectors have emerged as an important category of medications. These agents, such as sucralfate, act by forming a protective barrier over the stomach lining, shielding it from irritants and promoting healing. This dual action not only alleviates discomfort but also allows for the natural repair processes of the stomach to take place more effectively. The combination of acid blockers and mucosal protectors can offer a comprehensive approach to treating stomach diseases.

Recent studies have highlighted the potential benefits of combining these new acid blockers with mucosal protectors. This synergistic approach can lead to more effective management of symptoms and improved healing rates. Healthcare providers are increasingly recognising the importance of tailoring treatment regimens to individual patient needs, which can include the use of these innovative medications. As awareness grows, patients are encouraged to discuss the latest options with their healthcare professionals.

In conclusion, the development of new acid blockers and mucosal protectors represents a significant advancement in the treatment of stomach diseases. As these medications become more widely available, they offer hope for many individuals suffering from chronic gastrointestinal issues. Staying informed about these developments is vital for both patients and healthcare providers to ensure optimal management of stomach-related conditions.

Targeted H. pylori eradication

Targeted eradication of H. pylori, a bacterium linked to various stomach diseases, is essential for improving gastrointestinal health. This approach involves specific treatment regimens designed to eliminate the bacteria while minimising side effects. With rising antibiotic resistance, tailored therapy is becoming increasingly important in achieving effective eradication rates.

The most common treatment for H. pylori infection includes a combination of antibiotics and proton pump inhibitors (PPIs). These medications work synergistically to not only kill the bacteria but also reduce stomach acid, allowing for better healing of any associated ulcers. The precise duration and dosage of therapy can vary based on individual patient factors and local resistance patterns.

Recent studies have shown that personalised treatment strategies can significantly enhance eradication success. This may involve susceptibility testing to identify the most effective antibiotics for each patient. By taking these factors into account, healthcare providers can improve outcomes and reduce the likelihood of treatment failure.

In addition to medical management, lifestyle modifications play a crucial role in supporting targeted eradication efforts. Patients are encouraged to adopt a balanced diet, reduce stress, and avoid irritants such as tobacco and excessive alcohol. These changes can aid in recovery and help maintain a healthy stomach environment post-eradication.

Ultimately, the targeted eradication of H. pylori not only alleviates symptoms but also reduces the risk of developing serious complications like gastric cancer. Awareness and education about the importance of this treatment can empower individuals to seek appropriate medical advice and improve their overall digestive health.

Gastric microbiome research

The gastric microbiome plays a crucial role in the overall health of the stomach and the digestive system. Recent research has highlighted the complex communities of microorganisms residing within the gastric environment, which were once thought to be relatively sterile. These microorganisms, including bacteria, archaea, fungi, and viruses, interact with the host's immune system and can influence various physiological processes, including digestion and nutrient absorption.

One of the significant findings in gastric microbiome research is its relationship with stomach diseases, particularly gastric cancer and gastritis. Studies have shown that certain bacterial populations, such as Helicobacter pylori, can contribute to the development of these conditions. Understanding the dynamics of the gastric microbiome may open new avenues for preventative and therapeutic strategies in managing stomach diseases.

Moreover, the composition of the gastric microbiome can be affected by several factors, including diet, lifestyle, and antibiotic use. Research indicates that a diet rich in fibre and fermented foods can promote a healthier microbiome, whereas high sugar and processed food consumption might disrupt its balance. This highlights the importance of lifestyle choices in maintaining gastric health and preventing disease.

Another exciting area of research involves the potential for probiotics to modulate the gastric microbiome positively. Probiotics are live microorganisms that can confer health benefits when consumed in adequate amounts. Preliminary studies suggest that specific probiotic strains may help restore balance to the gastric microbiome, thereby reducing the risk of diseases like gastritis and improving overall stomach health.

In conclusion, the exploration of the gastric microbiome is a rapidly evolving field that holds significant promise for improving our understanding of stomach diseases. As more research is conducted, it is likely that we will uncover additional insights into how these microbial communities influence health and disease. Continued advancements in this area may lead to innovative approaches for diagnosis, treatment, and prevention of gastric-related conditions.

Non-invasive cancer screening methods

Non-invasive cancer screening methods are crucial in the early detection of stomach diseases, particularly gastric cancer. These methods aim to identify the presence of cancer without the need for surgical procedures or biopsies. By utilising advanced technologies and techniques, healthcare professionals can assess the risk and presence of cancer more safely and comfortably for the patient.

One prominent non-invasive method is the use of breath tests, which analyse volatile organic compounds in the breath that may indicate cancer. Studies have shown that certain biomarkers can be detected, allowing for early intervention. This approach is not only less invasive but also more accessible for many patients, potentially leading to increased participation in screening programmes.

Another significant technique is the application of imaging technologies such as ultrasound and magnetic resonance imaging (MRI). These methods provide detailed images of the stomach and surrounding organs, helping to identify abnormalities without the discomfort associated with endoscopies.

Their ability to visualise soft tissues makes them invaluable for diagnosing stomach diseases and monitoring changes over time.

Blood tests are also emerging as a vital tool in non-invasive cancer screening. Researchers are exploring the potential of specific blood markers that could indicate the presence of gastric cancer. These tests can be performed quickly and easily, offering a convenient option for patients and healthcare providers alike.

In summary, non-invasive cancer screening methods are transforming the landscape of stomach disease diagnosis. By focusing on comfort and accessibility, these innovative techniques are likely to enhance early detection rates and improve patient outcomes. As research progresses, the integration of these methods into routine screening practices may significantly reduce the burden of stomach cancer on patients and healthcare systems.

14

Detailed Briefing Document: The Essential Guide to Stomach Diseases

This briefing document provides a comprehensive overview of the stomach, its functions, common diseases, diagnostic tools, treatments, and future trends, drawing key information and direct quotes from "The Essential Guide to Stomach Diseases."

15

I. Anatomy and Physiology of the Stomach

The stomach is a complex, muscular, hollow organ crucial for digestion, located between the oesophagus and the small intestine. Its structure and function are intricately linked, involving both gross and cellular anatomy, hormonal regulation, acid secretion, and neural control.

A. Gross Anatomy

The stomach is divided into four main regions, each with a distinct role:

- **Cardia:** The entry point from the oesophagus, containing the lower oesophageal sphincter to prevent backflow. "The cardia is the section where the oesophagus connects to the stomach. This area is crucial as it contains the lower oesophageal sphincter, which prevents the backflow of stomach contents into the oesophagus."
- **Fundus:** A storage area for undigested food and gases, adaptable in shape.
- **Body:** The largest region, central for "mixing and churning food with gastric juices, which contain hydrochloric acid and digestive enzymes." This mechanical breakdown forms chyme.
- **Pylorus:** The distal end connecting to the small intestine, controlled by the "pyloric sphincter, which regulates the passage of chyme into the duodenum."

B. Cellular Structure

The stomach wall comprises four layers:

- **Mucosa:** The innermost layer, with specialized epithelial cells secreting gastric juices (hydrochloric acid and digestive enzymes) from gastric pits. "This layer is crucial for the initial stages of digestion."
- **Submucosa:** Rich in blood vessels, nerves, and connective tissue, supporting the mucosa and regulating secretions.
- **Muscularis:** Three layers of smooth muscle (inner oblique, middle circular, outer longitudinal) enabling powerful contractions (peristalsis) for mixing and propelling food.
- **Serosa:** The outermost protective layer, reducing friction with other organs.

C. Hormonal Regulation

Several hormones regulate gastric function:

- **Gastrin:** Stimulates gastric acid secretion and mucosa growth.
- **Ghrelin:** The "hunger hormone" produced in the stomach, signaling appetite. "Its levels rise before meals and decrease after eating, thus playing a pivotal role in meal initiation and energy balance."
- **Somatostatin:** Inhibits gastrin and other digestive hormones, balancing gastric function and preventing excessive acid secretion. Disruptions in this hormonal balance can lead to disorders like gastritis or peptic ulcers.

D. Acid Secretion and Protection

Gastric acid, primarily hydrochloric acid, is essential for breaking down food and killing harmful bacteria.

- **Secretion:** Regulated by neural and hormonal signals (e.g., gastrin, vagus nerve).

- **Protection:** The stomach protects itself with a thick **mucus layer** and **bicarbonate ions** to neutralize excess acidity, preventing damage and conditions like gastritis and ulcers. "The gastric mucosa, or stomach lining, secretes a thick layer of mucus that acts as a barrier against acid." Imbalances in acid secretion or protective mechanisms are central to many stomach diseases.

E. Neural Regulation and the Enteric Nervous System (ENS)

The **Enteric Nervous System (ENS)**, often called the "second brain," is an autonomous neural network within the GI tract.

- **Function:** Regulates digestion, muscle contractions, and enzyme secretion, influenced by food presence and chemical signals.
- **Interactions:** Influenced by the **gut microbiome** and connected to the brain via the **gut-brain axis**, demonstrating how stress and emotions can impact gut health. "This connection illustrates how stress and emotional states can influence gut health and vice versa."

16

II. How the Stomach Works in Digestion

A. Mechanical and Chemical Digestion

Digestion in the stomach involves:

- **Mechanical Digestion:** Physical breakdown of food through muscular contractions, mixing it with gastric juices.
- **Chemical Digestion:** Molecular breakdown of food by acids (hydrochloric acid) and enzymes (e.g., those breaking down proteins). These processes work in tandem, and inefficiency in either can lead to "incomplete digestion, causing discomfort and potential stomach diseases."

B. Stomach Emptying and Coordination with Small Bowel

The stomach gradually releases **chyme** into the small intestine, a process influenced by food type (e.g., high-fat meals slow emptying) and hormones (gastrin, cholecystokinin).

- **Complications:** Too rapid emptying (dumping syndrome) or delayed emptying (gastroparesis) can cause significant digestive issues.

C. Stomach's Role in Nutrient Absorption and Vitamin B12

The stomach is critical for activating enzymes and processing nutrients.

- **Vitamin B12:** The stomach produces **intrinsic factor**, a protein essential for vitamin B12 absorption in the intestines. "This binding is crucial because, without intrinsic factor, vitamin B12 cannot be adequately absorbed in the intestines, leading to potential deficiencies." Stomach diseases can impair intrinsic factor production, leading to B12 deficiency and related symptoms like fatigue and neurological issues.

17

III. Gastric Disorders - Symptoms and Signs

Common symptoms of stomach diseases include:

- **Dyspepsia (Indigestion):** Upper abdominal discomfort, bloating, nausea, fullness, caused by diet, stress, or underlying conditions like GORD or peptic ulcers.
- **Nausea/Vomiting:** Common responses to irritation, infections, or side effects of medications. Persistent vomiting can lead to dehydration.
- **Early Satiety:** Feeling full after consuming small amounts of food, often linked to gastroparesis, peptic ulcers, tumours, or hormonal imbalances.
- **Bloating and Belching:** Sensation of fullness and expulsion of gas.
- **Epigastric Pain:** Pain in the upper central abdomen (sharp, burning, or dull ache), indicative of gastritis, peptic ulcers, GORD, pancreatitis, or even cardiac issues. "Common causes of epigastric pain include gastritis, peptic ulcers, and gastroesophageal reflux disease (GORD)."
- **GI Bleeding:** Serious condition manifesting as:
- **Haematemesis:** Vomiting blood (bright red or coffee ground-like), indicating upper GI bleeding. "It is crucial for individuals experiencing these symptoms to seek immediate medical attention, as the underlying causes can be life-threatening."
- **Melena:** Black, tarry stools from digested blood, indicating bleeding higher in the GI tract.

18

IV. Gastritis and Inflammatory Conditions

Inflammation of the stomach lining:

- **Acute Gastritis:** Sudden onset, often from excessive alcohol, NSAIDs, or *H. pylori* infection.
- **Chronic Gastritis:** Develops gradually, due to prolonged irritant exposure, autoimmune disorders, or *H. pylori*.
- **H. pylori-associated Gastritis:** Caused by *Helicobacter pylori* bacteria, a leading cause of chronic gastritis, peptic ulcers, and increased risk of stomach cancer. "The presence of H. pylori can lead to chronic gastritis, which may subsequently increase the risk of peptic ulcers and even stomach cancer if left untreated."
- **Autoimmune Gastritis:** Immune system attacks gastric cells, leading to loss of acid and intrinsic factor production, often causing B12 deficiency.
- **Radiation and Caustic Injury:** Damage from radiation therapy or ingestion of corrosive substances, causing inflammation, ulceration, bleeding, or perforation.

19

V. Peptic Ulcer Disease (PUD)

Sores on the stomach or small intestine lining:

- **Gastric vs. Duodenal Ulcers:** Gastric ulcers are in the stomach lining, often causing pain shortly after eating. Duodenal ulcers are in the duodenum, more common in younger individuals, and pain appears a few hours after eating when the stomach is empty.
- **Pathogenesis:** Primarily caused by:
- ***H. pylori* Infection:** Disrupts the protective mucus layer.
- **NSAIDs:** Inhibit prostaglandin production, which protects the stomach lining. "Without adequate prostaglandins, the stomach becomes more susceptible to damage from its own acidic environment, leading to potential complications such as ulcers and gastritis."
- **Acid Imbalance:** Excessive acid production (e.g., in GORD).
- **Diagnosis and Red Flags:** Diagnosis involves patient history, physical exam, blood tests, endoscopy, and imaging. **Red flags** requiring immediate attention include "unintentional weight loss, persistent vomiting, or blood in stools."
- **Treatment:** Often a multifaceted approach:
- **Triple/Quadruple Therapy:** For *H. pylori*, combining a PPI with two or three antibiotics (sometimes bismuth).
- **Proton Pump Inhibitors (PPIs):** Reduce gastric acid production to

promote healing. "By decreasing acid secretion, PPIs help to create a more favourable environment for the stomach to heal, while also providing relief from discomfort and preventing further damage to the lining."

- **Lifestyle Modifications:** Balanced diet (avoiding spicy/acidic foods), physical activity, healthy weight, stress reduction.
- **Drug-Induced Damage:NSAIDs and Aspirin:** Inhibit protective prostaglandins, increasing vulnerability to acid, leading to ulcers and gastritis.
- **Other Drugs:** Antibiotics (disrupt gut flora), corticosteroids (increase acid, reduce mucus), certain antidepressants (SSRIs), and blood thinners can also damage the gastric lining.

20

VI. Functional and Motility Disorders

Conditions where stomach function is impaired without an obvious structural cause:

- **Functional Dyspepsia:** Symptoms like bloating, discomfort, and nausea without an identifiable organic cause. Linked to altered gastric motility, increased GI sensitivity, and psychological factors.
- **Gastroparesis:** Delayed gastric emptying, causing nausea, vomiting, bloating, and abdominal pain. Often associated with diabetes (nerve damage) or certain medications.
- **Rapid Gastric Emptying (Dumping Syndrome):** Food moves too quickly from the stomach to the small intestine, common after gastric surgery. Symptoms vary by phase: early (nausea, cramps, diarrhea) and late (dizziness, sweating, rapid heart rate due to blood sugar drop).

21

VII. Gastric Malignancies

Types of stomach cancer:

- **Gastric Adenocarcinoma:** Most common type, originating from glandular stomach lining tissue. Risk factors include chronic *H. pylori* infection, diet, smoking, and genetics. Symptoms are often vague, making early detection crucial.
- **Gastrointestinal Stromal Tumors (GISTs):** Unique tumours arising from interstitial cells of Cajal, often linked to KIT or PDGFRA genetic mutations. Symptoms can be absent or include abdominal pain, nausea, GI bleeding. Targeted therapies (e.g., imatinib) have revolutionized treatment.
- **Gastric Lymphomas:** Cancer originating in stomach lymphatic tissue, distinct from adenocarcinoma. Most prevalent is MALT lymphoma, often linked to *H. pylori* infection. Treatment may include *H. pylori* eradication.
- **Screening and Surveillance:** Regular screenings (e.g., **endoscopy**) and non-invasive tests (breath tests for *H. pylori*, imaging) are crucial for early detection, especially for high-risk individuals. "Early detection is crucial, as it can significantly improve treatment outcomes and overall prognosis."

22

VIII. Rare and Structural Stomach Conditions

- **Menetrier's Disease (Hypertrophic Gastritis):** Rare disorder with abnormal growth of stomach lining, forming large folds. Causes abdominal pain, nausea, vomiting, and can lead to nutritional deficiencies.
- **Gastric Polyps:** Abnormal growths on the stomach lining. Most are benign, but adenomatous polyps have a higher cancer risk. Symptoms are often subtle or absent.
- **Bezoars:** Accumulations of indigestible materials (hair, fibers, medications) in the GI tract, causing pain, nausea, vomiting, or obstruction.
- **Gastric Volvulus:** Life-threatening condition where the stomach twists on itself, obstructing the digestive tract and potentially cutting off blood flow. Requires immediate surgical intervention.
- **Congenital Conditions (e.g., Pyloric Stenosis):** Narrowing of the pylorus, common in infants, causing projectile vomiting and dehydration. Treated surgically.

23

IX. Bariatric Surgery and the Stomach

Bariatric surgeries modify the digestive system for weight loss.

- **Types:Gastric Bypass:** Creates a small stomach pouch connected directly to the small intestine.
- **Sleeve Gastrectomy:** Removes a large portion of the stomach, leaving a smaller, sleeve-shaped stomach.
- **Adjustable Gastric Banding:** Places an adjustable band around the upper stomach.
- **Mechanisms:** These surgeries limit food intake and/or reduce nutrient absorption, affecting appetite-regulating hormones.
- **Long-Term Effects and Nutritional Considerations:** Can lead to nutrient malabsorption and deficiencies, requiring careful dietary management and hydration.

24

X. Diagnostic Tools in Gastric Disease

- **Endoscopy (EGD):** A "pivotal diagnostic procedure" for direct visualization of the oesophagus, stomach, and duodenum, allowing for biopsy. Used for ulcers, tumours, inflammation.
- **Urea Breath Test:** Non-invasive test to detect *H. pylori* by measuring labeled carbon dioxide in breath after urea ingestion. "The urea breath test is a non-invasive diagnostic procedure used primarily to detect the presence of Helicobacter pylori..."
- **H. pylori Stool Antigen:** Non-invasive test detecting *H. pylori* antigens in stool, indicating active infection.
- **Gastric pH Monitoring:** Measures stomach acidity levels using a pH probe, helpful for GORD or acid overproduction.
- **Imaging (CT, Barium Meal):CT Scans:** Provide detailed cross-sectional images for tumours, inflammation, structural issues.
- **Barium Meal Studies:** Use barium contrast for X-rays to visualize stomach lining, helpful for ulcers, blockages, GORD.
- **Gastric Emptying Studies:** Assess the rate food leaves the stomach, diagnosing conditions like gastroparesis.

25

XI. Medications for Stomach Disorders

- **Proton Pump Inhibitors (PPIs):** Block proton pump to reduce gastric acid production, treating GORD, ulcers. Long-term use has potential side effects.
- **H2 Receptor Antagonists (H2 Blockers):** Inhibit histamine's action on H2 receptors, reducing gastric acid secretion. Used for GORD and ulcers.
- **Prokinetics (Domperidone, Metoclopramide):** Enhance gastrointestinal motility to alleviate nausea, vomiting, bloating. "These medications work by increasing the movement of food through the stomach and intestines..."
- **Sucralfate, Antacids, Mucosal Protectants:Sucralfate:** Forms a protective barrier over ulcers.
- **Antacids:** Neutralize stomach acid for rapid relief.
- **Mucosal Protectants:** Safeguard stomach lining, stimulate mucus/bicarbonate production.
- **Antibiotics for *H. pylori*:** Specific regimens (e.g., triple therapy: PPI + two antibiotics) to eradicate the bacteria, crucial for treating infections and preventing recurrence of ulcers and cancer.

26

XII. Lifestyle, Diet, and Mental Health

- **Role of Diet in Symptom Management:** A balanced diet can alleviate symptoms; spicy/acidic foods, caffeine, alcohol can exacerbate. Hydration, portion control, and meal timing are crucial.
- **Stress, Anxiety, and Functional Symptoms:** Emotional states significantly impact stomach health via the **gut-brain axis**, altering motility and microbiome balance. Can trigger/exacerbate conditions like IBS and functional dyspepsia. Stress reduction is vital.
- **Alcohol, Caffeine, and Smoking Effects:Alcohol:** Irritates stomach lining, increasing gastritis/ulcer risk.
- **Caffeine:** Stimulates gastric acid secretion, potentially aggravating reflux.
- **Smoking:** Weakens oesophageal sphincter, linked to ulcers, hinders healing.

27

XIII. Future Trends and Innovations

- **New Acid Blockers and Mucosal Protectors:** Ongoing development of improved PPIs and mucosal protectants for enhanced efficacy and reduced side effects.
- **Targeted *H. pylori* Eradication:** Personalized treatment strategies, including susceptibility testing, to combat antibiotic resistance and improve eradication rates.
- **Gastric Microbiome Research:** Exploring the complex communities of microorganisms in the stomach and their role in diseases like gastric cancer and gastritis, opening avenues for preventative and therapeutic strategies (e.g., probiotics). "Understanding the dynamics of the gastric microbiome may open new avenues for preventative and therapeutic strategies in managing stomach diseases."
- **Non-invasive Cancer Screening Methods:** Development of breath tests, advanced imaging (ultrasound, MRI), and blood tests for early and comfortable detection of gastric cancer.

28

FAQ

1. What are the main anatomical regions of the stomach and their functions?

The stomach is a muscular, hollow organ divided into four primary regions: the cardia, fundus, body, and pylorus. The **cardia** is where the esophagus connects, containing the lower esophageal sphincter to prevent backflow. The **fundus**, located above the cardia, serves as a storage area for undigested food and gases. The **body** is the largest region, crucial for mixing and churning food with gastric juices, breaking it down into chyme. Finally, the **pylorus**, at the stomach's distal end, connects to the small intestine and contains the pyloric sphincter, which regulates chyme release into the duodenum for controlled digestion and nutrient absorption. Understanding these regions is vital to comprehending stomach function and potential disease implications.

2. How does the stomach protect itself from the highly acidic environment it creates for digestion?

While essential for digestion and killing harmful bacteria, gastric acid can be corrosive. The stomach has robust protective mechanisms to prevent damage to its own lining. The primary defense is the **gastric mucosa**, which secretes a thick layer of **mucus** that acts as a physical barrier against acid. Additionally, **bicarbonate ions** are secreted to neutralize any excess acidity near the stomach lining. These protective layers and neutralizing agents are crucial in preventing conditions like gastritis and ulcers, which can occur if this delicate balance is disrupted.

3. What is the role of the Enteric Nervous System (ENS) in stomach function?

The Enteric Nervous System (ENS), often called the "second brain," is an extensive network of neurons embedded in the walls of the gastrointestinal tract. It can operate autonomously, independently of the central nervous system. The ENS is crucial for regulating digestion by coordinating muscle contractions (peristalsis) and controlling the secretion of digestive enzymes and hormones. It processes information about the gut's state and responds to stimuli like food presence. Disruptions in ENS neural regulation can lead to various gastrointestinal disorders, highlighting its fundamental role in stomach function and overall digestive health. The ENS is also influenced by the gut microbiome and communicates with the brain via the gut-brain axis, further emphasizing its complexity and importance.

4. What are the key differences between mechanical and chemical digestion in the stomach?

Mechanical and chemical digestion are two essential, complementary processes in the stomach. **Mechanical digestion** involves the physical breakdown of food through muscular contractions, or peristalsis, which churns and mixes food with gastric juices, reducing it to smaller particles and eventually a semi-liquid substance called chyme. **Chemical digestion**, conversely, involves breaking down food at a molecular level using enzymes and acids. In the stomach, hydrochloric acid activates digestive enzymes like pepsin, which begin to break down proteins into smaller peptides. Both processes are crucial for converting complex food into simpler molecules that can be absorbed, and insufficient mechanical digestion can hinder effective chemical digestion.

5. What are common symptoms of stomach disorders, and what are some "red flags" that indicate a more serious condition?

Common symptoms of stomach disorders include dyspepsia (indigestion with bloating, nausea, and fullness), nausea and vomiting, early satiety (feeling full after small amounts of food), and epigastric pain (pain in the upper central abdomen, which can be sharp, burning, or dull). Bloating and belching are also frequently reported.

Red flags that necessitate immediate medical attention as they may indicate a more serious problem include:

- Unintentional weight loss
- Persistent vomiting
- Blood in stools (melena, characterized by black, tarry stools, or hematemesis, which is vomiting blood that may appear bright red or like coffee grounds)
- Difficulty swallowing

Recognizing these severe signs is crucial for prompt diagnosis and intervention, as early detection often leads to better treatment outcomes for conditions like gastric cancer or GI bleeding.

6. What are the primary causes of peptic ulcers, and how are they typically treated?

Peptic ulcers, which can occur in the stomach (gastric ulcers) or the first part of the small intestine (duodenal ulcers), are primarily caused by three factors:

1. **Helicobacter pylori (H. pylori) infection:** This bacterium colonizes the stomach lining, leading to chronic inflammation and disrupting the protective mucus layer, making the lining susceptible to acid damage.
2. **Non-steroidal anti-inflammatory drugs (NSAIDs):** Prolonged use of NSAIDs like ibuprofen or aspirin inhibits prostaglandins, which are vital for maintaining the stomach's protective barrier, leading to increased vulnerability to acid.
3. **Acid imbalance:** Excessive stomach acid production or compromised protective mechanisms can contribute to ulcer formation.

Treatment typically involves a multifaceted approach:

- **Triple or Quadruple Therapy:** For H. pylori infections, a combination of a proton pump inhibitor (PPI) and two or three antibiotics (e.g., amoxicillin, clarithromycin, metronidazole, plus bismuth in quadruple therapy) is prescribed to eradicate the bacteria.
- **Proton Pump Inhibitors (PPIs):** These medications reduce gastric acid production, aiding in ulcer healing and symptom relief.
- **Lifestyle Modifications:** Avoiding irritants like alcohol, smoking, and certain foods (spicy, acidic, fatty) is crucial. Stress management and a balanced diet are also important for healing and preventing recurrence.
- **Mucosal Protectants:** Medications like sucralfate can form a protective barrier over ulcers, promoting healing.

7. How do common substances like alcohol, caffeine, and tobacco affect stomach health?

Alcohol, caffeine, and tobacco can significantly impair stomach health.

- **Alcohol** irritates the stomach lining, leading to inflammation (gastritis) and increasing the risk of ulcers, especially with heavy, regular consumption.
- **Caffeine** stimulates gastric acid secretion, which can exacerbate conditions like acid reflux or gastroesophageal reflux disease (GORD), particularly in sensitive individuals or with excessive intake.
- **Smoking (Tobacco)** weakens the lower esophageal sphincter, increasing acid reflux likelihood. It also elevates the risk of peptic ulcers and hinders the healing process of existing gastrointestinal issues.

Combining these substances can amplify their detrimental effects, overwhelming the stomach's defenses and leading to compounded symptoms like severe heartburn, nausea, and abdominal pain. Understanding these impacts is crucial for maintaining digestive health.

8. What diagnostic tools are commonly used to assess stomach health and diagnose gastric diseases?

A comprehensive diagnosis of stomach diseases often involves a combination of methods:

- **Endoscopy (EGD):** A flexible tube with a camera is inserted to visually examine the esophagus, stomach, and duodenum. It allows for direct visualization of abnormalities like ulcers or tumors and enables biopsies for tissue analysis.
- **Urea Breath Test and H. pylori Stool Antigen Test:** These non-invasive tests detect the presence of Helicobacter pylori infection. The breath test identifies carbon dioxide produced by the bacteria after ingesting urea,

while the stool antigen test detects bacterial proteins in a stool sample.

- **Gastric pH Monitoring:** A pH probe is used to continuously measure stomach acidity levels, helping diagnose conditions like GORD by correlating pH levels with symptoms.
- **Imaging Studies:Computed Tomography (CT) scans** provide detailed cross-sectional images to identify structural abnormalities, inflammation, or tumors.
- **Barium meal studies** involve ingesting barium contrast to coat the stomach lining, enhancing visibility on X-rays to detect ulcers, blockages, or reflux.
- **Gastric Emptying Studies:** These tests measure how quickly food leaves the stomach, primarily to diagnose conditions like gastroparesis (delayed emptying) or rapid gastric emptying (dumping syndrome).

These tools provide critical insights for accurate diagnosis, guiding appropriate treatment plans, and monitoring patient progress.

29

📚 Books

1. **Sleisenger and Fordtran's Gastrointestinal and Liver Disease***Editors: Mark Feldman, Lawrence S. Friedman, Lawrence J. Brandt*

- A comprehensive reference covering all aspects of gastric diseases with excellent detail on pathophysiology and clinical management.

1. **Textbook of Gastroenterology** – *Tadataka Yamada*

- In-depth explanation of gastric physiology, H. pylori, and acid-related disorders.

1. **The Stomach: Physiology, Pathophysiology, and Treatment** – *Editors: Horst Schulz, Mark Feldman*

- Focuses specifically on the stomach, with detailed chapters on gastric hormones, acid secretion, and protective mechanisms.

1. **Gastrointestinal Physiology** – *Leonard R. Johnson*

- Clear and focused coverage of stomach function, hormones, and the enteric nervous system.

1. **Schwartz's Principles of Surgery** – *F. Charles Brunicardi et al.*

- Great surgical perspective, including up-to-date bariatric surgery options and postoperative care.

30

📄 Key Peer-Reviewed Articles

1. **"Gastric Physiology and Helicobacter pylori: Basic Mechanisms and Clinical Relevance"***Clinical Microbiology Reviews, 2005*

- Excellent breakdown of H. pylori's impact on gastric function.

1. **"Gastrointestinal Hormones and Regulation of Gastric Acid Secretion"***Physiological Reviews, 2007*

- Reviews the interplay between gastrin, somatostatin, and histamine in acid secretion.

1. **"Role of the Vagus Nerve in the Regulation of Gastric Functions"***Autonomic Neuroscience, 2001*

- Detailed description of vagal pathways and their role in motility and secretion.

1. **"Nonsteroidal Anti-inflammatory Drugs and the Stomach"***The American Journal of Medicine, 2001*

- A classic article outlining NSAID-related gastric injury mechanisms.

1. **"Gastric Cancer: Epidemiology, Prevention, Classification, and Treatment"** *Cancer Treatment Reviews, 2013*

- Current data on types, risk factors, and therapies for gastric cancer.

1. **"Gastrointestinal Complications of Bariatric Surgery"** *Gastroenterology Clinics of North America, 2010*

- Thorough review of the risks, mechanisms, and long-term follow-up of bariatric surgery.

31

🌐 Trusted Websites

1. **American Gastroenterological Association (AGA)🔗** https://www.gastro.org

- Professional guidelines and patient information on all stomach-related diseases.

1. **International Foundation for Gastrointestinal Disorders (IFFGD)🔗** https://www.iffgd.org

- Patient-friendly resources on dyspepsia, gastroparesis, and GERD.

1. **National Institutes of Health (NIH) – NIDDK🔗** https://www.niddk.nih.gov

- Reliable information on gastritis, ulcers, and stomach cancer.

1. **UpToDate** *(subscription-based)*🔗 https://www.uptodate.com

- Clinically vetted, evidence-based articles for in-depth understanding.

1. **National Cancer Institute (NCI) – Stomach Cancer** 🔗 https://www.cancer.gov/types/stomach

- Information on gastric cancer staging, treatment, and clinical trials.

1. **ASMBS – American Society for Metabolic and Bariatric Surgery** 🔗 https://asmbs.org

- Reliable source for types, outcomes, and complications of bariatric surgeries.

www.ingramcontent.com/pod-product-compliance
Lightning Source LLC
LaVergne TN
LVHW090422210926
848480LV00002B/652
* 9 7 9 8 2 3 2 9 0 6 4 9 8 *